HEALTHY SOCIETIES

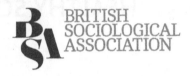

BRITISH
SOCIOLOGICAL
ASSOCIATION

What are the challenges shaping our lives today and in the future? At this time of social, political, economic and cultural disruption, this exciting series, published in association with the British Sociological Association, brings pressing public issues to the general reader, scholars and students. It offers standpoints to shape public conversations and a powerful platform for both scholarly and public debate, proposing better ways of understanding, and living in, our world.

Series Editors: Les Back, University of Glasgow, Nasar Meer, University of Edinburgh and Mónica G Moreno Figueroa, University of Cambridge

HEALTHY SOCIETIES

Policy, Practice and Obstacles

Graham Scambler

First published in Great Britain in 2024 by

Policy Press, an imprint of
Bristol University Press
University of Bristol
1–9 Old Park Hill
Bristol
BS2 8BB
UK
t: +44 (0)117 374 6645
e: bup-info@bristol.ac.uk

Details of international sales and distribution partners are available at
policy.bristoluniversitypress.co.uk

British Library Cataloguing in Publication Data
A catalogue record for this book is available from the British Library

ISBN 978-1-4473-7530-2 hardcover
ISBN 978-1-4473-7095-6 paperback
ISBN 978-1-4473-7096-3 ePub
ISBN 978-1-4473-7097-0 ePdf

Cover design: Lyn Davies Design
Bristol University Press and Policy Press use environmentally
responsible print partners.
Printed and bound in Great Britain by CPI Group (UK) Ltd,
Croydon, CR0 4YY

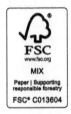

FSC
www.fsc.org
MIX
Paper | Supporting
responsible forestry
FSC® C013604

Contents

List of boxes

About the author

Graham Scambler is Emeritus Professor of Sociology at UCL and founding co-editor of the journal *Social Theory & Health*. He is also a Fellow of the Academy of Social Sciences, UK. His career has been committed to teaching and researching health and health care and he has written many books, chapters and journal articles on these issues.

Introduction

Health is a concept with many facets or dimensions. To a doctor it typically indicates an absence of signs and symptoms of disease. This overlaps with but by no means exhausts lay understandings. Acknowledging this, sociologists have conventionally distinguished between medical definitions of *disease* and lay interpretations of *illness*. Thus, it is possible for people to have a disease without defining themselves as ill, and conversely, for people to define themselves as ill without having a disease. We tend in fact to see ourselves as ill if our lives are disrupted in some way, either through troublesome symptoms that a doctor would recognise, or because through pain or impairment we cannot get on with our lives by going to work or by engaging in normal daily routines. For some, often those enjoying a degree of middle-class affluence and security, the criteria for good health are more ambitious, culminating in a wish for a positive sense of *wellbeing*. But health need not be confined to the properties of individuals. Populations and even societies are sometimes defined as healthy or otherwise.

The idea of a healthy population or society implies that it is somehow health-bestowing; and that it is inherently comparative, that is, healthy compared to *other* populations or societies. The criteria used in such cases vary widely, often encompassing data on life expectancy at birth, age-group mortality, health-related quality of life and access to health care services. Many of these measures treat populations, and even societies, as aggregates of individuals. Without denying the usefulness of studies that compare populations and societies in this way, it is a basic tenet of this book that societies and the social institutions that comprise them cannot be reduced to aggregates of individuals. Social institutions and what I shall term *social structures* do not admit of analysis in these limited and limiting terms.

What follows is the product of long-term frustration. There has accumulated a considerable literature on the health of populations around the globe and on the health care systems that serve those populations. While these accounts often include commentaries on the obstacles would-be reformers face in improving things, missing from many of them is an analysis of the role of impediments that have their tap roots in deep and abiding social structures. While passing mention is often now made of the salience of social structural considerations for health and health care, it is almost as if it would be rude to face up to the ramifications of this. It is a central theme of this book not only that the causal impact of social structures is of fundamental importance for the distribution of health and life expectancy and for the reach and effectiveness of health care systems, but that they play their part in inhibiting confronting this fact.

Given the importance of the concept of structure in what follows, it warrants some attention at the outset. The sociological literature abounds with definitions and with claims made on its behalf, and the arguments around it can become extremely complex. A good starting point is the observation that society precedes us. We are all born and socialised into pre-existing social structures or relations. These shape us without fully deciding our futures as people and as citizens: by our behaviours we reproduce existing relations or, more rarely, transform them. It can be said that our lives are structured without being structurally determined. The fact that we have some potential also to transform the social worlds we inhabit means that we have agency. But clearly agency can be either enabled by our structural circumstances or constrained by them. As we shall see, our precise point of entry into society matters a great deal. Culture, too, plays a significant part in who we become and what impact we have on events; and culture is also socially structured.

A good way of clarifying these early remarks on structure, agency and culture is by means of examples. Take the case of someone born into a working-class nuclear family on a mix of zero hours contracts and Universal Credit, struggling with the post-pandemic 'cost of living crisis' presently engulfing life in England: that is, a family hit simultaneously by low and declining incomes and significant rises in energy costs and rampant inflation in food and other basic goods. Now compare this set of natal circumstances with those of a child entering what is nominally the same social world but in this case one in which the new arrival is protected by the joint incomes of professional parents. It should come as no surprise that the former's prospects of emerging unscathed from the cost of living crisis are diminished relative to the latter. The term 'unscathed' here has a diverse multiplicity of strands, ranging from the realisation of educational, occupational and material ambitions to access to support systems and the enjoyment of good health and longevity. It was the American sociologist Robert Merton who first wrote of the 'Matthew effect', so named after the passage in the Gospel according to Matthew that cites Jesus: 'to anyone who has, more shall be given, and he will grow rich; from anyone who has not, even what he has will be taken away'. It refers in other words to the tendency for advantage to give rise to further advantage. Of course, there are statistical exceptions to this structured patterning of people's prospects, but as we shall see they are precisely that, *exceptions*. Moreover, underlying the social patterning that these vignettes exemplify is a set of social structures that make transforming the status quo very difficult and highly contested. These structures are rarely obvious: they are beneath-the-surface phenomena that in various combinations shape events on the surface, and the existence of which must be inferred from our empirical investigations of surface event patterns.

A good illustration of what is meant here comes from research on education and social mobility. It might seem obvious that success in school examinations is the key to future job and income security and wellbeing. But Bukodi and Goldthorpe's (2018) sophisticated programme of empirical research challenges this piece of common sense. What they found was that the barriers facing students from working-class backgrounds do not end if they make it into the examination room, or even if they get good results. What really matters is not 'equality of opportunity', which is what common sense and politicians emphasise, but 'equality of condition'. Notwithstanding a significant post-Second World War rise in the overall educational level of the British population, this has had very little effect in weakening the association that exists between individuals' class origins and their class destinations. To return to the contrast in the preceding paragraph between a child born into a hard-up working-class family and one born into an affluent professional family, the latter enjoys structural and cultural advantages that go far beyond the remit of the education system to address. As Bukodi and Goldthorpe insist, it is inequalities of condition that need addressing. It is an argument of resonance to health and health care as well as to education.

The focus of this volume is on health, and one myth that requires prompt debunking is that the health of a population is primarily a function of the nature of its health care system. This common-sense presumption is wide of the mark. The analogy with education should be apparent, though it can obviously not be pushed too far. One recent regional American estimate is that medical care accounts for only 10–20 per cent of the modifiable contributors to healthy outcomes for a population, though the authors readily admit that precise data are hard to come by, especially for cross-cultural comparisons (Hood et al, 2016). But if this estimate holds at least some water, then considerable causal salience must be accorded to *social determinants of health*, which the World Health Organization (WHO) defines as follows: 'the conditions in which people are born, grow, live, work and age. These circumstances are shaped by the distribution of money, power and resources at global, national and local levels' (World Health Organization, 2012). Behind this statement by the WHO lie enduring social structures and cultures that enable the agency of the few even as they constrain the agency of the many.

I shall argue that principal among the social structures impacting on both the health of the contemporary population of England and the nature, parameters and reach of the National Health Service (NHS) is *social class*. This is not to under-value important social structures such as gender and race or ethnicity, which will also feature; but I shall argue here that it is class that is pivotal for our understanding of the maldistribution of health and health care nationally and internationally through the multiple phases of capitalism since the 'long' 16th century and culminating in today's rentier capitalism. What I mean by class goes beyond the numerous proxies for class which have become standard tools for empirical research in the area and are often referred to as 'occupational class (or status)'. These proxies include the now largely defunct Registrar General's 'Classification of Occupations' and its replacement, the National Statistics Socio-economic Classification (NS-SEC) (latest version 2020). NS-SEC is in many respects an improvement on its long-serving predecessor. It purports to measure the employment relations and conditions of occupations, and as such it is an entirely appropriate tool for researching a wide range of social phenomena, including social mobility. I will contend, however, that NS-SEC is of limited use in any credible sociology of health and health care. This is in part because it carries a very real potential to deflect attention from social structural analysis, the more so given that most empirical researchers in the health field work with large secondary data sets, which means that they can only ask questions that can be answered from within the data set.

The concept of social class deployed in this text harks back to the pioneering theories of Marx and might properly be designated neo-Marxist. It is a concept that will be explored in some detail in the chapters that follow, but it will suffice here to insist that references both to a 'ruling class' and to 'class struggles' are still applicable, and that the distinction between capital ownership and wage labour remains pivotal, albeit within structural and cultural landscapes unanticipated by Marx a century and a half ago. It will be argued that the *maldistribution* of health and longevity especially cannot be understood or explained without factoring in relations of class. In a nutshell, a case will be made that a ruling class comprising a fraction of the 1 per cent identified by the Occupy Movement are now in a position to 'buy' enough political power to steer the state's economic, social and health policies in their interests, namely, towards the further accumulation of their capital; and that a largely unintended consequence of this is a deepening of what Bukodi and Goldthorpe (2018) presciently called inequalities of condition, a notion that travels well beyond the education system. It should already be apparent that identifying and examining the ruling class and its influence is not possible via the likes of NS-SEC. What research using NS-SEC does do, however, is provide us with clues about the nature and progeny of class relations and their deep and pervasive societal impacts, and, even more so, clues as to just how it is that macro-phenomena like class set in motion a chain of reactions that leads to the penetration of our skins and the impairment of our organs (Bartley, 2016).

5

The chapters that follow might well exercise different levels of appeal to different categories of reader. Many colleagues in epidemiology and public health will be familiar with much of the material in Chapters One and Two for example, and those in health policy with the contents of Chapters Three and Five; but this is not to deny their explicit sociological slants. The analyses to be found in Chapters Seven and Eight – on planetary health and warfare, respectively – may surprise some readers, but embody sets of issues that are critical for any credible concept of a healthy society. The theoretical chapters towards the end of the book are more obviously sociological but it is hoped that these might interest health researchers and practitioners seeking ways of linking their knowledge and experience to macro-aspects of social order and social change. The concluding chapter, Chapter Twelve, is more specifically addressed to sociologists of health and health care and confronts them – 'us' – with a series of challenges to confront in a fractured society in an increasingly fractured world. Although much of the text is focused on England/the UK, the ramifications have a wider relevance.

Chapter One notes that notions of health, illness and disease vary by time and place, as do systems of healing. They are, in other words, moveable feasts. But all of us are born and will eventually die. Historical and comparative data on international rates and causes of mortality are outlined and discussed. These establish a set of parameters at the beginning of the book. The point is made, however, that our present concepts and practices might have developed differently, are constantly evolving and will inevitably change in the future. Chapter Two focuses on social determinants of health in general and health inequalities in particular. The evidence for entrenched inequalities and their deepening in the 21st century is documented. Means of addressing them are critiqued for their lack of ambition. An alternative way of explaining health inequalities in terms of structural and cultural mechanisms is outlined. Special attention is paid to the 'greedy bastards hypothesis' (GBH), which asserts that the main cause of the growing maldistribution of health and longevity rests with those members of a ruling class of 'nomadic' transnational bankers, major shareholders and CEOs whose executive decisions filter down to impact negatively on those with the fewest material and psychosocial resources.

Chapter Three switches attention from the structural causes of health inequalities to those responsible for the collapse of the NHS. Class relations and the GBH again play a prominent role, as does the changing dynamic between class and state. It is shown how the NHS has been undermined by stealth via a calculated political strategy. It is a process of undermining that Chomsky characterised by the formula: first underfund to, second, create public dissatisfaction, then, third, send for the private sector to 'rescue' services.

Chapter Four focuses on the fractured society that rentier capitalism has delivered and the structural and cultural impediments to achieving a healthy society. One contention is that structural relations, such as social class, gender, race or ethnicity and age, that are important causes of widening health inequalities and threats to the integrity of the NHS, also function as obstacles to meaningful social and institutional reform in our 'fractured society'. Disability, sexuality and geographic space in the form of region, community and neighbourhood are also important. Cultural factors of salience include the collapse of universal or general narratives around progress and change and their substitution by individualised and fragmented narratives based on identity.

Chapter Five introduces the notion that the COVID-19 pandemic acted as a kind of 'breaching experiment', throwing a harsh spotlight on the inequalities and inequities that characterise English society. In fact, the pandemic has demonstrably broadened the cracks and fissures of what I have elsewhere defined as our 'fractured society'. The pandemic also afforded opportunities for highly questionable government policy-making 'on the hoof', at its extremes involving clear cases of chumocracy, cronyism and corruption. The emergence of the fractured society, with all its consequences for population health and the health care system, is shown to be a product of the post-1970s transition from welfare state capitalism to financialised or rentier capitalism.

A key focus has been on the changing situation in England. In some ways this is typical of changes elsewhere, and in other ways not. In Chapter Six a case is made that the analysis of *any* nation state qua healthy society must be extended as a matter of urgency to incorporate analyses of global relations. Reference is made both to shifts in the global economy of significance for health and health care beyond the English experience and to the contemporary concerns around climate change attributed to the 'age of the Anthropocene'. Chapter Seven extends the discussion to consider the links between humans and nature in the form of planet Earth. Recognising that nature is not external to and independent of humans in the Anthropocene, it dwells on the changing relations between our species and its habitat and the ramifications of this shift for health and health care. Chapter Eight focuses on another phenomenon of continuing salience for health across the globe, namely, war.

In Chapters Nine and Ten the importance of constructing credible theories of intra- and intersocietal order and change is stressed. Key parameters for such a theoretical project are spelled out. Critically, these go beyond merely extending Anglo-Saxon, European and Australasian sociological theories to apply them to 'other or non-Western societies' and to global relations. The outline of a new paradigm is offered, incorporating perspectives from, for example, neo-Marxist world systems theory and post-colonial, feminist and environmental sociologies.

In Chapter Eleven a case is made that the analysis of *any* nation state qua healthy society must be extended as a matter of urgency to incorporate analyses of global and planetary relations. Reference is made both to shifts in the global economy of significance for health and health care and to the contemporary concerns around climate change attributed to the 'age of the Anthropocene', or of the 'Capitalocene'. The discussion is extended in this chapter to consider the links between humans and nature in the context of conceiving and delivering effective policies and practices for health and health care in the 21st century. In doing so it confronts the structural and cultural obstacles to its implementation and specifies the perils of failing to do so. In Chapter Twelve the threads of the thesis built through Chapters One to Nine are pulled together, and the potential for realising the transformations discussed is assessed. The book closes with an analysis of sociology's rightful engagement with these issues in anticipation of a probable perfect storm of health-related crises.

ONE

The healthy society

It is something of a cliché that just as we as individuals are born into a ready-made society, so this same society is, in many fundamental respects, a product of prior societal forms. How best to interpret the past has given rise to a discrete area of study known as 'hermeneutics'. Are we to understand past societies in terms of the frames of reference of those inhabiting them at the time? Or deploying the frames of reference available to us in the present? Or can we as historians or social scientists develop frames of reference that somehow transcend these past–present divides? What is unquestionable is the omnipresent requirement that these hermeneutic quandaries and the sensitivity and restraints they demand are understood and factored into historical-social enquiries. As will become clear, what we might call 'health problems' have inevitably varied by time and by place. Less resistant to capture are variations in life expectancy: after all, *all* humans are born, live their lives, and then die. The problems with data on life expectancy hinge on their paucity and validity. It is only relatively recently that data, globally and by continent and nation state, have become available, permitting comparative analyses; but even these data sets admit of variation due to inter- and intranational differences in data collection and processing.

Box 1.1 offers a summary of historically evolving types of society. What this does is help position and facilitate analyses of social order and change and their ramifications for population health and health care. But two qualifications are necessary. First, the whole business of 'periodising' history is problematic and can easily mislead the unwary: there is always a mix of continuity and change. I have used the phrase 'pendulum paradox' to allude to this issue. It tends to be sociologists who look for and trade on the patterning of events and want to theorise about social order and social change. Historians on the other hand prefer to focus on events and sequences of events. When the pendulum swings towards sociology, critiques typically emphasise the complexity of events; and when it swings towards history, critiques complain of an unnecessary curtailment of explanatory ambition. The second qualification echoes an argument forcefully made by Graeber and Wengrow (2021), namely, that only too often we see previous societies not only in light of our own but as more 'primitive' or less sophisticated than our own. In short, we have a teleological view of history, as if the past was destined to culminate in an improved present. The extensive research of Graeber and Wengrow gives the lie to this trite presumption (causing the paradox pendulum to swing back towards complexity). But notwithstanding these qualifications, the contents of Box 1.1 constitute a sociologist's

---

Box 1.1: A chronology of historical types of society

From the beginning of the Neolithic revolution, occurring from 8000 to 3000 BC, socio-political evolution encompassed four principal stages:

1. *Bands* – small nomadic groups of up to a dozen hunter-gatherers; democratic and egalitarian (close to Marx's 'primitive communism').
2. *Tribes* – similar to bands except more committed to horticulture and pastoralism; 'segmentary societies' comprising autonomous villages.
3. *Chiefdoms* – autonomous political units under permanent control of paramount chief, central government with hereditary, hierarchical status arrangements; 'rank societies'.
4. *States* – autonomous political units; centralised government supported by monopoly of violence; large dense populations characterised by stratification and inequality.

Fully fledged agrarian states appeared around 3000 BC. These displayed a number of core characteristics and remained the predominant form of social organisation until around 1450 AD. These core characteristics can be summarised as follows:

- a division of labour between a small landowning (or controlling) nobility and a large peasantry; this was an exploitative division backed by military force;
- the noble–peasant relationship provided the principal axis in agrarian societies: it was a relationship based on production-for-use rather than production-for-exchange;
- differences of interest between nobles and peasants, but not overt 'class struggle';
- societies held together not by consensus but by military force;
- societies relatively static and unchanging: there was a 4,500-year incubation period prior to the advent of capitalist states.

The transition to capitalism took place in the 'long sixteenth century', that is, between 1450 and 1640. Marx saw this transition as of major significance, noting three vital characteristics of the new capitalist system:

- private ownership of the means of production by the *bourgeoisie*;
- the existence of wage labour as the basis of production;
- the profit motive and long-term accumulation of capital as the driving aim of production.

It is customary to discern reasonably distinct stages of capitalism. Thus a transition to 'merchant capitalism' typically dates from 1450 to 1640, followed by a period of consolidation and solidification, characterised by slow, steady growth between 1640 and 1760. The year 1760 is often cited as a marker for a switch to 'industrial capitalism', which is itself often divided into stages:

1. *Early industrial*, 1760–1830: textile manufacturing dominated by Britain.
2. *Liberal*, 1830–1870: railroads and iron dominated by Britain and later the USA.
3. *Liberal/Early Fordist*, 1870–First World War: steel and organic chemistry, with the emergence of new industries based on producing and using electrical machinery, dominated by the USA and Germany.
4. *Late Fordist/Welfare*, First World War–1970: automobiles and petro-chemicals, dominated by the USA.
5. *Financial*, 1970 onwards: electronics, information and biotechnology, plus global finance, dominated by the USA, also Japan and Western Europe.

Source: Adapted from Scambler (2018)

'ideal typical' device for charting changing types of society: the Weberian concept of an ideal type recognises the importance of analysing types of phenomena, which is part and parcel of doing sociology, but also admits of empirical complexity and variation.

'Guesstimates' based on a paucity of surviving artefacts suggest that life expectancy at birth for hunter-gatherers eking out a life-course of unpredictability, subsistence and hardship scarcely exceeded 20 years or so, though those who made it through the especially hazardous initial few days, weeks and months doubtless added on a good few more years. Estimations of life expectancy at birth after the Neolithic revolution coalesce around 30 years in all regions of the world, and this figure holds good throughout premodern times; that is, up to the unfolding of early industrial capitalism in the West. It should be emphasised, however, that surviving childbirth and infancy has always been critical. Historian Ian Mortimer (2014: 3) puts it well in his study of change from 1000 to 2000:

> Even in the Middle Ages, some men and women lived to 90 years of age or more. St Gilbert of Sempingham died in 1189 at the age of 106; Sir John de Sully died in 1387 at 105. Very few people today live any longer than that. True, there were comparatively few octogenarians in the Middle Ages – 50 per cent of babies did not even reach adulthood – but in terms of the maximum lifespan possible, there was little change across the whole millennium.

From the start of the 19th century, life expectancy at birth began to increase in early industrial societies, though it remained low in the rest of the world. In other words, this period saw the advent of a growing gap between the neophyte industrial societies and the pre-industrial world. This gap has remained, though no society in the world currently has a lower life expectancy than those with the highest life expectancy in 1800. Since 1900 the global average life expectancy has more than doubled and is now above 70 years. But the inequality of life expectancy is still large: in 2019 the country with the lowest life expectancy was the Central African Republic with 53 years, 30 years lower than that in the highest, Japan.

Disease patterns over time

Among contemporary Western commentators a consensus has emerged on the existence of three historical *disease patterns*. Considering these briefly at the outset will give us a context and a set of parameters for the theses to be introduced and developed later. As already mentioned, before the Neolithic revolution people lived as hunter-gatherers without any form of settled agriculture. In fact, this period of history covered most of the evolution of humans as a species. A best guess on the basis of admittedly scant surviving artefacts is that for those who survived into adulthood the pre-eminent causes of death were probably the issue of environmental hazards, including hunting accidents, malnutrition and exposure. More information is available on causes of death in the more settled states based on agriculture that existed from 3000 BC onwards as bands, tribes and chiefdoms became peripheral. The development of cereals allowed for more mouths to be fed in these states, which in turn led to increased population densities. But at the same time the restricted cereal-based diet likely lessened people's resistance to infection. Hence the emergence of a range of infectious diseases as primary causes of mortality. The four main modes of transmission were: (i) airborne (for example, tuberculosis); (ii) waterborne (for example, cholera); (iii) food-borne (for example, dysentery); and (iv) vector-borne (for example, plague and malaria). Most dramatically, the Black Death that swept through Europe in 1348 decimated populaces, accounting for an astonishing quarter of the total European population. Spread by fleas carried by black rats its last visit to Britain was in 1665; after this it died out as black rats were displaced by brown rats less prone to infest human settlements.

It is now widely accepted that the historically rapid acceleration of longevity in the second half of the 19th century in countries such as Britain was precisely due to the declining significance of the infectious diseases. The evidence is that improvements in mortality occurred at different times for different age groups. In Britain the initial improvement occurred in the 5–14 age group around 1860. Infant mortality fell steadily from 1900. In 1900, one-quarter of all deaths in the population occurred in the first year of life: this is one reason why so many of our Victorian forebears gave birth more often than have succeeding generations. But by the end of the century this had declined from a quarter to 1 per cent. Mortality rates for the 15–44 age group improved through the course of the 20th century, if with interruptions from the influenza epidemic of 1918 and the two world wars. Improvements for those aged 45–54 also began at the start of the century. For those aged 55–74 mortality declined from the 1920s. The decline for those aged over 75 began after the Second World War; and for even older age groups the most marked improvements in mortality have taken place since the 1970s (Fitzpatrick and Chandola, 2000).

Why did the infectious diseases lose salience in countries like Britain from the era of liberal capitalism onwards? Several specific theories have been advanced. The first focuses on a decline in the virulence of the organisms responsible for these diseases. A second hypothesis is that there occurred an enhanced genetic human resistance to infection due to Darwinian selection processes. A third stresses a reduction in human exposure to the infectious organisms, for example through the reduced contamination of water and food supplies. Finally, it has been claimed that an important role should be accorded increased human resistance to infection through improved nutrition and general fitness. As so often, it is not a case of picking one of this quartet to the exclusion of the others. Nor is it possible to insist on an order of priority across all the major infectious diseases or all societies. There are firm grounds, however, for maintaining that the first two theories (a decline in the virulence of the organisms, and enhanced genetic resistance due to natural selection) can largely be discounted because the decline across the infectious diseases occurred over too short a time and across all the major diseases.

There is strong evidence supporting the fourth theory (increased human resistance through improved nutrition and general fitness). Nutritional intake improved partly because of innovative agricultural techniques and partly through the more efficient transportation of produce under liberal capitalism. Also relevant was the fact that the 19th century witnessed an unprecedented increase in real wages and hence in standard of living. This is not to deny a role also for the third theory (reduction in exposure to infection). John Snow's iconic experimental removal of a pump handle in London's Soho, in the process affirming cholera's status as a waterborne disease, heralded the 19th-century emergence of a far-reaching public health movement. Measures were subsequently taken to prevent the contamination of supplies of drinking water by sewage, with the result that gastroenteric diseases were under control by the beginning of the 20th century, dramatically reducing infant mortality in the process. The sterilisation of milk and its more hygienic transportation was another innovation, as was improved food hygiene in general. In sum, it seems clear that most of the – in fact, dramatic – decline in death rates occurring in countries like Britain by the time of the Second World War can be attributed to a broad category of environmental factors, though other phenomena such as the decline in the birth rate, the reduced demand for food and housing, improvements in the quality of housing and better personal hygiene also played their part. Importantly, the decline in mortality from most of the infectious diseases occurred *before the introduction of effective treatments and immunisation*, which is not of course to downplay their importance when they did become available from the 1930s onwards.

In countries like Britain the primary causes of death associated with the decline of the infectious diseases and enhanced longevity, as liberal/early Fordist capitalism transmuted into late Fordist/ welfare capitalism, were chronic and degenerative conditions such as cardiovascular disease and the cancers. These brought new and different challenges for governments, welfare systems and for health and social care. Lofland (1978) has distinguished between the generalised displacement of premodern 'quick' by modern 'slow' dying. As well as reflecting a shift from a high incidence of mortality from acute disease to a high incidence of mortality from chronic or degenerative disease, this also reflected pervasive shifts: from a low to a high level of medical technology; from a late to an early detection of potentially fatal diseases; from a simple to a more complex definition of death; and from a generally passive orientation to death to a curative and interventionist emphasising of the prolongation of life.

Several lessons can be taken from the extensive literature on disease patterns and causes of death briefly represented here. First, it is readily apparent that the most telling critical interventions during Western liberal/early Fordist to late Fordist/welfare capitalism trespassed far beyond direct applications of medical and clinical expertise. Social and environmental factors played vital roles in each transition in disease pattern, and among such factors is that panoply of 'social determinants of health' defined in the Introduction. Even allowing for the pivotal role of the public health movement in the decline of mortality from the infectious diseases, it remains the case that the prevailing pattern of mortality by time and place is, at least in part, a reflection and function of prevailing patterns of social organisation. It has been claimed by some that Adam Smith's 'invisible hand' of capitalism itself holds the key, but this leaves open the question of which of capitalism's numerous properties are conducive to population health (and which are not).

A second observation is that the differences in the primary causes of death (still) vary significantly between low-income and high-income countries. As Box 1.2 shows, while six of the top ten causes of death in low-income countries involve communicable diseases, this is true of only one in high-income countries.

Box 1.2: Leading causes of death globally across different types of society in 2019

Leading causes of death: globally	Leading causes of death: low-income countries
Ischaemic heart disease	Neonatal conditions*
Stroke	Lower respiratory infections*
Chronic obstructive pulmonary disease	Ischaemic heart disease
Lower respiratory infections*	Stroke
Neonatal conditions*	Diarrhoeal diseases*
Trachea, bronchus, lung cancers	Malaria*

Alzheimer's disease and other dementias

Diarrhoeal diseases*

Diabetes mellitus

Kidney diseases

Leading causes of death: lower middle-income countries

Ischaemic heart disease

Stroke

Neonatal conditions*

Chronic obstructive pulmonary disease

Lower respiratory infections*

Diarrhoeal diseases*

Tuberculosis*

Cirrhosis of the liver

Diabetes mellitus

Road injury

Leading causes of death: high-income countries

Ischaemic heart disease

Alzheimer's disease and other dementias

Stroke

Trachea, bronchus, lung cancers

Chronic obstructive pulmonary disease

Lower respiratory infections*

Road injury

Tuberculosis*

HIV/AIDS*

Cirrhosis of the liver

Leading causes of death: upper middle-income countries

Ischaemic heart disease

Stroke

Chronic obstructive pulmonary disease

Trachea, bronchus, lung cancers

Lower respiratory infections*

Diabetes mellitus

Hypertensive heart disease

Alzheimer's disease and other dementias

Stomach cancer

Road injury

Colon and rectal cancers

Kidney diseases

Hypertensive heart disease

Diabetes mellitus

Note: * Indicates communicable diseases

Source: Adapted from World Health Organization (2020)

We shall see that it is too simple to infer from this that 'less developed' societies *lag behind* for want of implementing effective social and health policies. Indeed, writing in terms of degrees of development, with its implication that today's Western liberal-to-financial capitalist regimes offer a necessary and well-trodden route towards or even the endpoint of the 'good society' is profoundly misleading. It needs to be acknowledged, too, that the causes of death outlined here are premised on modern Western 'scientific' theories, models and classifications of disease. In other cultures this paradigm is often less pervasive. And nor is contemporary Western sociology's distinction between *lay theories* of 'illness' and *professional medical theories* of 'disease' as clear-cut or compelling across cultures. Indeed, even understandings of death itself can and do vary. In some South Pacific cultures, for example, it is believed that life vacates a person's body intermittently during episodes of sleep or illness; thus a person can be said to 'die' many times. The Truskese of Micronesia maintain that life ceases at the age of 40, so that at the age 40 a person is, in effect, dead. At this point people withdraw from community activities and prepare to depart even as they are treated as dead by their communities. What this means is that although it is helpful to establish certain parameters for comparing the health of populations through comparisons of mortality rates, extending to causes of death, this should be the starting point for sociologists, not the endpoint.

A third comment concerns the nature of those social and environment factors that are critical for population health. Although inter- and intra-societal health inequalities are the focus of Chapter Two, it is important to acknowledge here a pivotal distinction between health inequalities and health inequities. The latter is a subset of the former and refers to those inequalities it is within our collective capacity to address and ameliorate. In practice, it is not always easy to distinguish between the two. For example, while it has long been accepted practice to contrast the 'givens' of human nature and the external environment with our human capacity to plan and engineer change, this is now under attack. Genetic engineering can be deployed to modify human nature, and the birth of the era of the Anthropocene has forced us to accept that our species is not only part of, but is actively shaping, the external environment. What Beck (1982) when delineating the 'risk society' called the 'boomerang effect', that is, the propensity in modern society for human-made risk to bounce back to affect the whole species, is now widely recognised. While in principle this recognition might increase our opportunities to better understand and to remedy existing health inequalities, the obstacles in our path are intimidating.

A final observation is that concerns about sustaining and improving the health profile of countries such as Britain has knock-on effects on the profiles of other countries. The data encapsulated in Box 1.2 bear eloquent testimony to this. The focus on creating a healthy British society has rested in the past, and in many respects continues to rest, on a dominant and exploitative relationship with other semi-peripheral and peripheral countries in the world or global concatenation of states. In other words, there are typically contradictions between the pursuit of population health at home and its pursuit in less well-placed countries overseas. Just how and why this is will become clearer when the social determinants of health are analysed in detail in later chapters.

The healthy society and the sociological task

It is a key theme in this volume that sociology's established agenda for studying people's health requires amending. With a handful of honourable exceptions, it has typically been concerned with the health of people within a particular modern Western country, and this without much by way of reference to two-way or international influences. This is not a problem per se, but it becomes problematic if the sociological community *as a whole* limits its ambitions in this way. There are two points to be made. First, it has become necessary to adopt a global perspective, even in relation to single-country-based studies. As will be made clear, this does *not* simply mean extending the reach of accepted Western paradigms. And second, there is a strong case for accepting a role for what is sometimes called 'normative sociology'. I have elsewhere addressed this by extending Burawoy's (2005) four types of sociology by appending two further types (Scambler and Scambler, 2015; Scambler, 2018). The resulting six types are represented in Box 1.3, together with characterisations of the sociologists and modes of engagement involved.

Box 1.3: Six sociologies and their representatives and logics

Sociologies	Sociologists	Modes of engagement
Professional	Scholar	Cumulative
Policy	Reformer	Utilitarian
Critical	Radical	Meta-theoretical
Public	Democrat	Communicative
Foresight	Visionary	Speculative
Action	Activist	Strategic

Source: Adapted from Scambler and Scambler (2015)

Much of the existing literature on the people's health comes into the category of professional sociology, and its scholars are committed to building incrementally towards an ever more comprehensive understanding and explanation of what is happening and why. It is, or should be, the type of sociology that provides the bedrock for sociological analysis. But it has too often been found wanting in the sociology of health and health inequalities, not least through its 'colonisation' by social epidemiology and consequent overriding commitment to positivistic or 'multivariate' enquiry. I have argued that while the discipline of epidemiology is rightly oriented to prediction in the sometimes-urgent service of public health policy and practice, sociology ought rather to be geared to painstaking causal explanation (Scambler, 2018). While multivariate analysis has yielded many interesting and useful findings, it has too often been regarded as the endpoint of, rather than a resource for, causal explanation. Variables are not structures. It is the identification and explication of enduring social structures as causal mechanisms that should be the primary focus for sociology's scholars. These structures, much like gravity in the fields of physics and astronomy, cannot be observed directly, so their existence and causal powers must be inferred from quantitative and qualitative empirical investigations (including those relying on multivariate analysis). This is a theme running through the present volume and is explored in more detail in Chapter Two.

Policy sociology's reformers are motivated by a desire to improve people's lot, occasionally via wholesale reform packages but more typically via piecemeal social engineering. As with the scholars of professional sociology, policy sociology's reformers can play an important role within and beyond the discipline. My main critique of their performance in the field of health and health care is their poverty of ambition. Far too many punches are pulled by reformers constrained by the pursuit of funding opportunities and by an eagerness to be taken seriously by 'people with influence' who often have a vested interest in the status quo. As a result, more attention is paid to exhorting citizens-cum-consumers to stop smoking, reduce alcohol consumption and abandon fast food outlets than to the increasingly transnational and pathogenic for-profit corporations that foster precisely these risk behaviours.

Critical sociology sustains the reflexive analyses of radicals who scrutinise the nature of the sociological project itself, so as the preceding paragraphs suggest there is a case for seeing this whole book as an example of critical sociology in practice. The democrats representing public sociology share sociology's findings and ruminations with a view to informing and 'educating' deliberation in the public sphere. There is perhaps a too-ready presumption that the engagement with civil society and the public sphere will inevitably impact positively on the quality, salience and effectiveness of policy and practice, but the truth is often more complex. When Richard Wilkinson and Kate Pickett (2009) published their widely read paperback entitled *The Spirit Level*, in which they argued that the more unequal a more 'developed' society, the more social problems – from criminal, extending to homicidal and suicidal propensities, to health disparities – accrue and impact, they were subject to a sustained ideological assault by powerfully placed antagonists who were beneficiaries of existing inequalities. The very real obstacles facing sociology's democrats are one reason why I was prompted to append two further types of sociology to Burawoy's quartet.

The visionaries representing foresight sociology are oriented to the consideration of alternate futures, that is, optimal or better ways of organising our affairs. One objection to a sociological project that trades in 'concrete utopias' is that it turns sociology from a professional or scientific to a normative exercise. Interestingly, few practitioners seem troubled by presumptions that a healthy society is *better than* a less healthy or an unhealthy one; nor do they baulk at a *moral imperative* to reduce health inequalities. I shall contend later in this contribution that normativity is inscribed in the sociological project and that we fail as a community if we do not recognise this. Moreover, in the closing chapters I directly address *what must be done* if we are to pursue a healthier society in Britain, a project now necessarily framed in the context of a healthier world and planet.

Action sociology's activists are the 'enforcers' of public sociology: they openly engage in political debate with a view to combatting calculated ideological neglect, dismissals or misrepresentations of sociological research. There exists an undoubted tension between the logics or modes of engagement of public and action sociology. While the former is rooted in a communicative orientation towards a rational consensus, the latter is based on a strategic or instrumental approach to victory in debate, policy and practice. This is an uncomfortable if unavoidable tension. But, if sociology is to amount to something more than an anodyne discipline submissive to institutional pressures and vested interests, it is a tension with which we must live and reconcile ourselves.

I have argued that no individual sociologist can do justice to all six types of sociology. Rather, it is as a community that we must ensure that all bases are covered. As the arguments of this text unfold, the roles and importance of foresight and action sociology in particular will become clearer. The challenges facing advocates for population health in the rapidly maturing age of the Anthropocene are immense. This age of the Anthropocene might perhaps more accurately, or precisely, be termed the age of the 'Capitalocene', denoting a geopolitics of capitalism as a world-ecology of power and re/production in the 'web of life'. These issues are theorised in Chapter Eight and various ways of tackling the structural and cultural obstacles to change are set out in Chapters Nine and Ten.

TWO

Social conditions and health inequalities

As the WHO definition in the Introduction made clear, the concept of 'social determinants of health' covers a complex and politically challenging range of phenomena. In this chapter I first document the extent of present health inequalities in this country before discussing how these have changed over time and appraising rival explanatory theories. The emphasis will then switch to professional and policy sociologists' culpable neglect of social structure in general and class relations in particular.

Health inequalities have been defined and measured in various ways, for example in terms of life expectancy, healthy life expectancy, long-term health conditions, access to formal care via the health care system, the quality of care received, behavioural risks to health, or wider factors such as income or housing. Consider first, life expectancy. This is closely related to people's socio-economic circumstances. The Index of Multiple Deprivation, which is based on factors like people's levels of income, employment, education and local levels of crime, is sometimes used to summarise the extent of people's deprivation within an area. In England, there is a strong relationship between deprivation and life expectancy. In 2017–19 women living in the least deprived 10 per cent of areas could, at birth, expect to live to 86.4 years, whereas women in the most deprived areas could expect to live to 78.7 years, a gap in life expectancy of almost eight years. For men, this gap was even wider, with a difference of 9.4 years between the life expectancy for those in the least deprived 10 per cent of areas (83.5 years) and the most deprived 10 per cent of areas (74.1 years). For any given level of deprivation, life expectancy in the north of England is lower than in the south of England. These inequalities have widened in recent years (King's Fund, 2022).

The King's Fund also comments on healthy life expectancy. In 2017–19, people living in the least deprived areas could expect to live almost two decades longer in good health than those in the most deprived areas. People in the most deprived areas spend approximately a third of their lives in poor health, twice the proportion spent by those in the least deprived areas. This means that the former spend, on average, a far greater part of their already far shorter lives in poor health. Geographical inequalities are once again prominent. In 2017–19, healthy life expectancy at birth for women in the north-east of England was 59.0 years, compared to 65.9 years for women in the south-east, a gap of 6.9 years. For men, this gap was 5.9 years.

Deaths are defined as avoidable if they could have been avoided by timely, effective health care ('treatable mortality'), or by broader public health and preventive interventions ('amenable mortality'). In 2019, nearly 140,000 – or around one in five – deaths in the UK were deemed avoidable. In England in 2019, women in the most deprived areas were 3.5 times more likely to die from an avoidable cause than those in the least deprived areas. Long-term conditions are a major cause of poor quality of life. In England, people in lower socio-economic groups are more likely to have long-term health conditions, and these conditions tend to be more severe than those experienced by people in higher socio-economic groups. Deprivation also increases the likelihood of having more than one long-term condition at the same time; on average, those in the most deprived fifth of the population develop multiple long-term conditions ten years earlier than those in the least deprived fifth. The data available on mental health are more patchy, but there is evidence that demand for mental health services is higher in more deprived communities, and that between 2010 and 2017 suicide rates among the most deprived decile were consistently around double the rates among the least deprived decile. More than 80 per cent of the homeless report having a mental health problem, and in 2019 people in this group were 14 times more likely than those in the general population to die by suicide. Asylum seekers and refugees were also at increased risk of experiencing depression, post-traumatic stress disorder and other anxiety disorders.

Analyses like this from the King's Fund that focus on links between deprivation and mortality and morbidity are more common than studies of health differentials related to individual socio-economic status (SES). One study by Ingleby and colleagues (2021), however, found that health inequalities are as strongly related to individual SES as to area-level deprivation. They conclude that poor outcomes are likely to be a product of 'both community and individual influence'. The Office of National Statistics (ONS) (2022) has analysed data from the 2021 Census for England and Wales and published estimates of life expectancy by individual socio-economic position using the National Statistics Socio-economic Classification (NS-SEC). As mentioned in the Introduction, NS-SEC is often understood and deployed as a proxy measure of social class. It assigns people to classes on clear criteria, namely the extent of job security; the presence of a career structure with opportunities for promotion; incremental pay increases; autonomy in relation to work schedule; authority over the work of others; and whether pay is by monthly salary or weekly or hourly. The basic divisions are between those who employ other people and exercise general control and authority over them; employees who sell their labour and find themselves under the control of employers in the process; and the self-employed, who experience neither (Bartley, 2016). Bartley summarises NS-SEC as follows:

- **Class 1**: *higher managerial and professional occupations* (including employers in large firms, higher managers and professionals, whether they are employees or self-employed).
- **Class 2**: *lower managerial and professional occupations and higher technical occupations*
- **Class 3**: *intermediate occupations* (clerical, administrative, sales workers with no involvement in general planning or supervision but high levels of job security, some career prospects and some autonomy over their own work schedule).
- **Class 4**: *small employers and own account workers*

- **Class 5**: *lower technical occupations*
  (with little responsibility for own planning work), lower
  supervisory occupations (with supervisory responsibility but no
  overall planning role and less autonomy over work schedule).
- **Class 6**: *semi-routine occupations*
  (moderate levels of job security, little career prospects, no pay
  increments, some degree of autonomy over their own work).
- **Class 7**: *routine occupations*
  (low job security, no career prospects, closely supervised
  routine work).

An additional category of 'Unclassified' includes the long-term
unemployed, those who have never worked, students, and
occupations inadequately described.

The ONS found that male life expectancy at birth in 2012–
16 was highest among higher managerial and professional
occupations (83.6 years), five and a half years longer than
routine occupations (78.1 years), and nine years longer than
males in the Unclassified category (74.5 years). Female life
expectancy at birth in 2012–16 was also highest in NS-SEC
Class 1 (85.5 years), four years longer than NS-SEC Class 7
(81.5 years), and over five and a half years longer than the
Unclassified category (79.8 years). In a study of adult self-rated
general health using data from the 2001 Census, Drever and
colleagues (2004) found a pronounced gradient in rates of 'not
good' health among people in different NS-SEC classes. The
rate for people in Class 7 was more than double that for people
in Class 1: 95 per 1,000 and 37 per 1,000, respectively. Health
inequalities were larger for men than for women, with the
greatest gap among people in Class 1.

What these studies and many others in the same mould produce
is incontrovertible evidence of marked and persisting health
inequalities whether analysed in terms of area-based community
or individual 'class-based' characteristics. Triggered by Marmot's
pioneering studies of British civil servants, it has frequently been
found that health inequalities are not just apparent in comparisons
between those 'at the top' of measures like NS-SEC and those 'at
the bottom', but that they show a fine-grained 'social gradient'
(see Marmot, 2006). The accumulation of these data over time has

led to a series of rival explanations. The 'Black Report' provided a seminal synopsis of these (Black et al, 1982). Its authors considered four possible explanations:

- the 'artefact' explanation asserted that neither class/socio-economic group nor health are easily measured and that the apparent link between the two might merely be a function of measurement decisions;
- the 'social selection' explanation claimed that health exerts a causal effect on class/socio-economic position rather than the other way round (that is, poor health leads to downward social mobility);
- the 'material/structural' explanation holds that material deprivation and hardship and a paucity of resources lead to poor health (that is, via low-income, substandard housing, and so on);
- the 'cultural/behavioural' explanation maintains that poor or impaired health is a function of engagement in risk behaviours such as smoking, bad eating habits, sedentary lifestyles, and so on, which are in turn embedded in particular cultures or subcultures.

While not dismissing any of the quartet, Black and his colleagues offered an evidence-based ranking of their relative importance. First was the materialist/structural; second the cultural/ behavioural; third the social selection; and fourth the artefact. Subsequent research has refined rather than demurred from Black's conclusions. For example, it has been convincingly argued that material/structural and cultural/behavioural factors are more closely related than was thought hitherto. People who struggle most with shortages of material resources are those most inclined to engage in so-called risk behaviours for health, in part because they have less access to health-bestowing goods, options, neighbourhoods and services, and in part too because such behaviours can afford a measure of compensation for impoverished lifestyles.

Since Black's comprehensive account, the artefact explanation has largely been laid to rest and explanations of health inequalities have tended to coalesce and cluster under three headings. There is a continued emphasis, first, on material factors; second, on behavioural and cultural factors; and third, on psychosocial factors. These have been extensively reviewed and I can be brief here since my critique takes off from their common limitations (see Bartley (2016) for a comprehensive summary of the literature). There is no questioning the continuing salience of material factors. As Black reported a generation ago, it is an approach that ranges widely over phenomena such as levels of wealth and income, the levels of toxicity and safety of work environments, the extent of job security, the quality of housing, and so on. Bartley has argued that material factors are most effectively studied over the whole life-course. Behavioural and cultural factors have also been extensively investigated since Black. They generally cover not only the patterned consumption of food, drink (especially alcohol) and cigarettes, but also the degree of use of preventive medical services and of immunisation, contraception and antenatal care. Bartley maintains that longitudinal studies of behaviours pertinent to health suggest that such behaviours account for around a third of the observed socio-economic differences in morbidity and mortality. It should be emphasised once more, however, that people's 'individual' behaviours are anchored not just in their culture but in their social and economic circumstances. As for the study of psychosocial factors, its advocates argue for the generally neglected causal role of 'psychosocial risk factors' such as work autonomy and social support. Wilkinson (1996) contends that income inequality leads to social fragmentation and dislocation, and hence to a collapse of social networks, reciprocity and trust. In short, 'social capital' is diminished, which is itself injurious to health and wellbeing.

There is merit in and empirical support for each of these approaches, though my task here is to show the sociological limitations they share. Consider the causal import Wilkinson attaches to income inequality (his 'relative income hypothesis'). Income inequality has certainly increased in Britain since the 1970s. It surged in particular under Thatcher in the 1980s and Britain is currently in pursuit of the USA as one of the most unequal among so-called 'developed' societies (it is second only to Lithuania as the most unequal society in Europe (Brewer, 2019)). Coburn (2000) has presciently objected to the Wilkinson hypothesis on the grounds that it uses income as its starting point, also that it subsequently accords priority to psychosocial pathways, with loss of social cohesion and diminution of trust providing the mechanisms linking high rates of income inequality with diminished health and longevity. Coburn laments the absence of any reference to social order and social stratification here. There has been an overwhelming socio-epidemiological tendency, he maintains, to focus on the possible social-psychological mechanisms through which social factors might be tied to health rather than on examination of the basic causes of inequality and health (Coburn, 2000). The offerings of socio-epidemiologists require deepening. In a later contribution, Coburn spells this out:

> People with high SES [socio-economic status] do indeed live longer than those with less. SES, however, is a mere ranking of people according to income, educational attainment or occupational position. It reflects standards of living generally, and because these standards are related to many different types of disease, it is a good correlate of health status. But SES is itself a result of class forces. The nature of the capitalist class structure, and the outcome of class struggles, determine the extent and type of socio-economic inequalities in a given society, and the socio-economic inequalities in turn shape the patterns of health – and of health care. But while many theorists of the social determinants of health proclaim an interest in the basic determinants of health and health inequalities, much of their literature omits any consideration whatever of the political and class causes of SES and the SES-health relationship. When they speak of analysing the 'causes' of disease, they seldom go far enough up the causal chain to confront the class forces and class struggles that are ultimately determinant. (Coburn, 2009: 44)

While it might be possible to construct a partial defence of this foreshortened analysis on the part of socio-epidemiologists committed to short-term policy interventions, it is inexcusable for sociologists necessarily operating on larger canvases.

The missing fraction of the 1 per cent

Britain remains a class-divided society, notwithstanding its multiple structural and cultural transmutations from the 'long sixteenth century' to today's rentier capitalism. And its contemporary class structure is inadequately addressed by classifications of socio-economic groups or statuses, even by more sophisticated versions like NS-SEC. I have elsewhere castigated the 'absence' from these various proxies for class of those whose highly concentrated ownership of capital buys more power from the state in post-1970s rentier capitalism than could possibly have been foreseen during the post-Second World War 'babyboomer' era of welfare state capitalism (Scambler, 2018). The less than 1 per cent that comprise the current incarnation of what John Scott (1991) called the 'ruling class' are able to hide in proxy classifications. My counter argument to sociologists overly inclined to socio-epidemiological research can be articulated via what I have called the 'class/command dynamic'. This will have resonance throughout subsequent chapters so warrants a fuller explication at this point. At its core are the twin assertions: (i) that a hard core of the capitalist executive class (those I term 'capital monopolists') can now buy more influence over policy-making from the power elite at the apex of the apparatus of the state than hitherto; and (ii) that this is causally decisive for the social maldistribution of health and longevity documented earlier. These claims are nestled within a broader picture of the structural and cultural relations of rentier capitalism.

Just as contemporary class relations must not be subsumed under proxy measures such as NS-SEC, so they must not be displaced by in-fashion representations of elite theory. This is not to deny a professional sociological role for either, but it is to resist their usage to nudge aside a proper consideration of class and class divisions. Scott (2008: 34) invites us to resist using 'economic elite' and 'capitalist class' interchangeably, however tempting. We must retain the elite concept, he contends, 'as this is the only basis on which the dynamics of power can be clearly understood'. My qualification is that throughout the phases of capitalism it is class that underpins the distribution and exercise of economic over political power. Analyses of economic and political elites should not stand in for or sidestep considerations of class. The class/command dynamic rests on the premiss that during post-1970s financialised or rentier capitalism, 'objective' class relations have extended their sway (directly) over the command relations of the state, and therefore (indirectly) over people's lives, even as 'subjective' class relations have diminished in salience. Sayer (2005) makes a similar point more eloquently when he insists that we must acknowledge the coexistence of 'identity-neutral' and 'identity-sensitive mechanisms'. He goes on to regret the tendency in recent research on inequality to focus on the latter to the near exclusion of the former. However convenient for contemporary neoliberal governments, 'identitarian politics' is no substitute for class-based politics.

Elsewhere Sayer (2015) usefully distinguishes between relations of class and those of gender and race. It is a pivotal distinction for this volume. While it is primarily sexism and racism that deliver inequalities of gender and race, class differences would persist even if the upper and middle classes were entirely respectful of the working class. This is because class prejudice, 'classism', is more a response to economic inequality than a cause of it. Enduring sexism and racism, on the other hand, would have a considerable impact on gender and race relations. He continues:

> Neoliberals – New Labour for example – can appear quite progressive about gender, race, sexuality, disability and condemn those who discriminate against people on these grounds. Unsurprisingly, the elephant in the room is economic inequalities or class difference. Though it never admits it, neoliberalism is a political-economic movement that seeks to legitimate widening economic inequalities and defend rentier interests above all others. Rentiers can live off others regardless of their gender, race, sexuality and so on. (Sayer, 2015: 170; see also Scambler, 2022)

This is not of course to diminish the importance of enduring inequalities of gender, race and so on. In fact, these inequalities typically preceded the advent of capitalism. *Capitalism has throughout its history run along gendered and racialised furrows even as it ploughed up and replanted those of class.* The emphasis on class will inform much of what follows. This is manifestly *not* to deny the merit of 'intersectionalist' approaches; but it is my limited if overriding aim here to re-address and re-appraise the nature of what I contend is the prepotent structural linkage between class and the domains of health and health care in contemporary society.

How are the capital monopolists and their class allies – the latter comprising what Byrne and Ruane (2017) call a 'concierge class' – the primary driver of Britain's worsening health inequalities? The context is provided in Box 2.1, which reproduces Byrne and Ruane's comparison of employment relations in the era of the welfare state with those in the age of the rentier economy.

Box 2.1: The principal differences in employment relations and taxation systems in industrial and post-industrial capitalism

Industrial employment relations and taxation system	Post-industrial employment relations and taxation system
Keynesian/Beveridge mode of regulation	Post-industrial/consolidation state mode of regulation
Industrial workforce approaching half of total workforce	Primarily service sector workforce; industrial workforce less than 15% of total
Full employment with frictional unemployment	Disguised unemployment (for example, extension of higher education; early retirement); underemployment
Job security and substantial worker rights	Flexible labour – spread of precarious employment, limited worker rights
Employer-borne risk and responsibilities to workforce	Transfer of risk to workers – use of zero hours contracts and forms of self-employment
Large public sector and devalorised labour	Declining public sector as proportion of all employment and recommodification of labour

Relatively high trade union membership	Low trade union membership
Relatively high wages	Lagging wages and spread of low wages; heavy reliance on wage subsidy
Strong protections for workers in public sector	Workers in public sector exposed to market competition
Status and protection for professionals	Extension of Fordism into professional work and proletarianisation
High top rates of income tax	Relatively low top rates of income tax
Relatively strong link between national insurance contributions and benefits received	Weak link between national insurance contributions and benefits received
Higher corporation tax rates	Lower corporation tax rates
Avoidance and evasion practices which do not catastrophically compromise the taxation system	Avoidance and evasion practices which catastrophically compromise the taxation system
Strong and independent tax collection authorities	Weakened tax collection authorities strongly influenced by corporate lobbying

Source: Byrne and Ruane (2017) [reproduced with permission]

The contemporary employment relations summarised here translate into a surge in job insecurity and material and material-related inequality which has been motivated above all else by the self-serving strategic behaviour of the capital monopolists. We can set aside for a moment the regressive easing of the personal and corporate tax burdens on the 1 per cent, a form of symbolic violence with which the four leading accountancy firms in Britain are complicit, and focus instead on other sequelae of capitalist monopolistic influence. The enhanced profits accruing to the few are attained at the price of further disadvantaging the many, and this is achieved via the decimation of trade union rights and the statutory safeguards protecting wage labour, the spread of free and cheap labour by means of internships, outsourcing and benefit cuts, each of these being falsely presented as a programme of rational austerity measures needed to address what is actually a growing deficit. This profiteering on the part of the less than 1 per cent kills people. (Campaigners such as Virchow and Engels were spot on.)

Precarity and the mushrooming of zero hours contracts, have become institutionalised in Britain, even as they demonstrably sap the health and longevity of those most affected. The advent of COVID-19, as Chapter Four will reveal, has served only to underline the structural contribution of the class/command dynamic to the social determinants of health. It was my anger at the widespread sociological neglect of the causal power of this dynamic that led me to the nomenclature of the 'greedy bastards hypothesis' (hereafter, perhaps even more graphically, the 'GBH'). The GBH asserts that growing health inequalities in the UK, as elsewhere, are *above all else* the unintended consequences of the self-serving decision-making of transnational financiers, major shareholders and CEOs: the sick and dying poor are collateral damage resulting from corporate profiteering.

Developing the concept of the GBH and its applicability, I have suggested that the idea of capital or 'asset flows' is fruitful. These are the means by which the class relations that the GBH represents impact – via the command relations of the state – on health and longevity. They are the 'media of enactment' of class relations. Seven empirically warranted types of asset flow can be distinguished:

• *Biological or body assets* can be affected by class even prior to birth. Low-income families, for example, are more likely to have low-birthweight babies, and low-birthweight babies carry an increased risk of chronic disease in childhood (possibly in part through 'biological programming').
• *Psychological assets* yield a general capacity to cope extending to what is often now termed 'resilience'. In many ways the 'vulnerability factors' that Brown and Harris (1978) found reduced working-class women's capacity to cope with those life events pertinent to the onset of clinical

depression are class-induced interruptions to the flow of psychological assets.

- *Social assets* or 'social capital' refer to aspects of social integration, networks and support.
- *Cultural assets* or 'cultural capital' are typically generated through processes of primary and secondary socialisation and can, in Britain's public schools for example, engender a special kind of fruitful 'belonging'. They encompass formal educational opportunities and attainment. Early class-related arrests to the flow of cultural assets can have long-term ramifications for jobs, income levels and therefore health.
- *Spatial assets* have been shown to be significant for health via area-based studies. Areas with high mortality tend to be areas with high rates of net out-migration; and it is often the better qualified and more affluent who exercise the prerogative to relocate.
- *Symbolic assets* stand for social status or 'honour' and have been shown to impact on people's health via their (sense of) their social position relative to that of significant others in their reference groups.
- *Material assets* signal the notion of 'relative deprivation' due to impoverishment and meagre standard of living. The relevance of material assets for health and longevity has long been established for all that the mechanisms linking low and falling incomes to health remain much debated.

Unsurprisingly, the notion of flows has gained little traction in the socio-epidemiological community given the problems it generates around systems of measurement oriented to multivariate analysis, even in longitudinal studies. But to my mind it fits the bill well. Each of the health-related asset flows identified here is consonant with the research literature: their causal relevance for health status and longevity has been established. Moreover, and crucially, each allows both for fluctuations in flow and for compensation between flows. It is obvious, for example, that an unexpected redundancy can drastically reduce the flow of material assets, cutting income and possibly leading to a threat of eviction from rental housing. But it is also possible for a degree of compensation to occur if there are strong flows of other health-bestowing assets, such as biological, psychological or social assets. Similarly, weak flows of biological, psychological or social assets might be mitigated by a strong flow of material assets. It should be noted that empirical research suggests that strong and weak flows tend to cluster together: typically, an individual will experience an accumulation of *either* strong flows *or* weak flows. A clustering of weak flows in infancy or early childhood can predict impaired adult health. Marmot (2006) also found that people's 'subjective' readings of their asset flows can have an impact on their health independently of the 'objective' – in principle at least, measurable – strength or weakness of flows.

Summarising the thrust of the class/command dynamic and the GBH at this juncture, rentier capitalism's realignment of class and state has led to a surge in wealth and income inequality made possible by a reinvigoration of class-based exploitation and state- or command-based oppression. This is pivotal for any credible sociology of health inequalities. Paradoxically, as I will argue, it also helps explain why such a 'credible sociology' remains marginal and spurned. There are now strong constraints around building academic careers via the metrics of funding revenue attained and publishing productivity. The endlessly replicated statistical associations linking socio-economic classifications and alternate proxies for class with health and longevity, leading for some to the idea of a social gradient, bear eloquent and irresistible testimony to the existence of real relations of class and to their causal efficacy: class as a social structure 'must' exist for the socio-epidemiological yield to be as strong and consistent as it is (Scambler, 2018).

Structure, culture and agency

The emphasis so far has been on neglected aspects of class as a social structure. In this section I touch on the salience of both culture and agency for health and longevity. Discussions of health inequality post-Black have rightly insisted that culture, and indeed agency, are structured, without being structurally determined. But the advent of financial or rentier capitalism has been accompanied by a discernible cultural shift towards 'cultural relativism'. As Lyotard (1984) argued, a handful of singular,

Western, Enlightenment-oriented *grand* narratives (for or against capitalism and often hinging on ideas of progress and the good society) have been displaced by a multitude of rival pick-and-mix *petit* narratives (largely focused on consumerism and identity). This has left the neoliberal worldview largely free from effective competition. Each *petit* narrative typically presents as an accessible 'ideology', allegedly leaving consumers free to choose and buy their way into their own personal worlds and identities. This shift, it should be noted, also represents a usurpation of the classical sociological notion of ideology. Ideology no longer specifically refers to a conveniently distorted worldview designed to disguise and provide cover for vested interests, but to *any* worldview. Contemporary culture has been 'relativised' or 'postmodernised', becoming in the process expedient for the class/command dynamic in that it denies the possibility of constructing rationally compelling *grand* narratives antithetical to the status quo. It is little wonder that with this cultural transition people's sense of self has become more detached from class as an objective or value-neutral mechanism. In other words, even as class now exercises *more* influence over people's material wellbeing, it provides *less* fuel for the construction of their identities. This does not mean, of course, that people's identities, including their sense of who they are, is irrelevant to their behaviour or their health. Just as this volume is not antithetical to intersectionalism, so it does not eschew the salience of identity for health; however, the primary descriptive and explanatory foci remain those concerned with objective and subjective aspects of class.

Agency is necessarily informed by structure and cultural recipes but does not reduce to them. Although we tend to tread in the deeply marked footsteps left by class, gender, race and so on, we are never entirely stripped of our freedom to change route and think and act independently. What Margaret Archer (2007) terms the 'internal conversations' that we routinely hold with ourselves mediate between the society that shapes us and our free will. *But* the neoliberal ideology that presently 'rationalises' rentier capitalism, together with a superfluity of *petit* narratives promoting identity-formation via consumption, have given rise to 'identitarianism', or the displacement of traditional *grand*-narrative based right-versus-left politics by a *petit* narrative based individualistic identity politics which, although itself salient for health and health behaviours, is also functional for the status quo. Identitarianism caricatures agency by offering the illusion of a greater latitude for decision-making than actually exists.

What implications do these preliminary snapshot comments on culture and agency have for health inequality in Britain? The main point to stress is that they have facilitated an insistent government rhetoric on the overriding importance of individual choice and, a companion notion, individual responsibility. When the Black Report was published it was quietly and speedily 'buried' by Thatcher's Minister for Health, Patrick Jenkin, in the hope that it would remain largely unread. Rather than prioritise the material/structural causes of poor health and reduced life expectancy, as Black commended, the government opted to prioritise cultural/behavioural causes. In later years this has transmuted into a government privileging of *lifestyle*, a facet of the newly emerging culture-ideology of 'lifestyle politics'. There is very little, it seems, that cannot be accommodated in this broadest of broad categories. The benefit for government in focusing on personal behaviour and lifestyle is that it allows for a transfer of overall responsibility for health from government to individual citizens. Poor health becomes a product of poor decision-making. This married well with Thatcher's assertion that 'there is no such thing as society'. Society for her was a misleading and inappropriate way of describing an aggregate of individuals (and their families). Moreover, the proper exercise of personal responsibility for one's own health was to be extended in the post-Thatcher years from a focus on cultural/behavioural issues such as smoking, diet, alcohol consumption and exercise to encompass material/structural phenomena such as employment, pay levels and housing. As we shall see in the next two chapters, economic, social and health policies have all come to be designed and appraised in part against the criterion of 'behavioural conditionality'; that is, they require people as citizens to demonstrate a moral worthiness to qualify for state services and help. Severe sanctions against those deemed to have failed to exercise due responsibility include health-damaging measures such as compulsory job-seeking, benefit cuts and the explicit rationing of health and social care.

At this point it is appropriate to introduce another sociological concept, that of the 'stigma/deviance dynamic'. Stigma here refers to a falling foul of social norms of *conformance*, while deviance refers to offences against norms of *compliance*. Stigma announces the *shame* deriving from the possession of an 'ontological deficit' (that is, failure as imperfection); and deviance involves the *blame* consequent on a 'moral deficit' (that is, failure as culpability). The stigma/deviance dynamic asserts that in the age of rentier capitalism 'blame has been heaped on shame' (Scambler, 2018a, 2020). Stigma, in short, has been 'weaponised' as deviance. This has allowed governments to cut services and avenues of support by sanctioning and punishing rather than helping people, for example for problems deriving from dis-abilities or disturbances of mental health: non-conformance has been widely recast as non-compliance. This stigma/deviance dynamic helps account for the ease with which the class/command dynamic has taken effect. To the extent to which the public buys into it, it helps smooth the path to further capital accumulation on the part of the capital monopolists and their allies. These two dynamics are important, too, for any consideration of how to tackle health inequalities.

In his *Fair Society, Healthy Lives (The Marmot Review)*, published in 2010, Marmot and colleagues outlined six policy objectives for reducing health inequalities: give every child the best start in life; enable all children, young people and adults to maximise their capabilities and have control over their lives; create fair employment and good work for all; ensure a healthy standard of living for all; create and develop healthy and sustainable places and communities; and strengthen the role and impact of ill-health prevention. Box 2.2 shows how the World Health Organization (WHO) has elaborated on items like these with a global framework mind.

Box 2.2: Recommendations from the WHO on social determinants of health

1. Daily living conditions

(a) A comprehensive approach to early child development, building on existing child-survival programmes and extending interventions in early life to include social/emotional and language/cognitive development.

(b) Sustained investment in rural development, addressing policies of exclusion that lead to rural poverty, landlessness and displacement of people from their homes; urban governance and planning.

(c) Economic and social policy responses to climate change and other environmental degradation taking into account health equity.

(d) Full and fair employment and decent work as a central aim of national and international social and economic policy-making; safe, secure and fairly paid work, year-round work opportunities, and a healthy work-life balance for all; improved working conditions for all workers in order to reduce exposure to material hazards, work-related stress, and health-damaging behaviours.

(e) Comprehensive social-protection policies that support an income level conducive to healthy living for all.

(f) Specifically with regard to the health sector, the Commission calls for the building of universal health care systems oriented around primary health care.

2. Inequitable distribution of power, money and resources

(a) Place responsibility for action on health and health equity at the highest level of government, and ensure its coherent consideration in all policies.

(b) Adjust the health sector as appropriate – include social determinants in the policy and programmatic functions of health ministries' stewardship role in supporting a social determinants approach throughout government.

(c) Strengthen public financing for action on social determinants; increase international financing for health equity, and coordinate increased finance by means of a framework for acting on social determinants.

(d) Reinforce the primary role of the state in providing basic services essential to health (such as water and sanitation) and regulating goods and services with a major impact on health (such as tobacco, alcohol and food).

(e) Address gender bias in the structures of society – in laws and their enforcement, in the way organisations are run and interventions designed, and in how a country's economic performance is measured.

(f) Reaffirm commitment to addressing sexual and reproductive health rights and rights universally.

(g) Empower all groups in society through fair representation in decision-making about how society operates, particularly in relation to its effect on health equity, and create and maintain a socially inclusive framework for policy-making.

(h) Enable civil society to organise and act in a manner that promotes and realises the political and social rights affecting health equity.

3. Monitoring the problem and interventions

(a) Ensure that routine monitoring systems for health equity and social determinants are in place locally, nationally and internationally.

(b) Invest in generating and sharing new evidence on how social determinants influence population health and health equity, and on the effectiveness or otherwise of measures to reduce health inequities through action on social determinants.

(c) Provide information about social determinants to policy actors, stakeholders and practitioners, and invest in raising public awareness.

Source: Adapted from World Health Organization (2008)

If the class/command and stigma/deviance dynamics have any explanatory purchase in relation to health inequalities in Britain (and in other kindred societies), it is immediately apparent that it is one thing to highlight the policies needed to reduce these inequalities, and quite another to implement them. The primary causes – structural, cultural and agential – of the health inequalities identified earlier precisely constitute the primary obstacles to tackling them. Recalling the study of social mobility by Bukodi and Goldthorpe (2018) cited in the Introduction, it is equality of 'condition' rather than that of (mere) 'opportunity' that is paramount. This takes us back to a key source of my frustration with the unwitting colonisation of so much of the sociology of health inequalities by social epidemiology. Many published studies in the field make little mention of class relations other than by proxy, let alone of capitalism, for all that it has become somewhat customary to conclude accounts with a knee-jerk reference to the explanatory salience of macro-social structural factors. In Chapters Three and Four the relevance of the analysis sketched in this chapter for the evolution and current state of health care in Britain and for the deeply flawed response to COVID, respectively, is further elaborated.

The items in Box 2.2 represent a general and wide-ranging strategy for addressing the global problem of obstinate health inequalities and inequities. It is even more apparent that the distance to travel globally in the face of recalcitrant structures, cultures and agential constraints is even more challenging than it is in Britain. I return to the global dimension of population health in Chapter Six. But there are two axiomatic points to emphasise at this juncture. The first is that what is continually omitted from the informative and aspirational series of national and international Marmot/WHO reports is *any consideration of how we get from where we are to where they recommend we end up.* There is a paradox here. 'Insiders' like Michael Marmot are listened to and politely sidelined, while 'outsiders' – of which I am unashamedly one – are simply ignored. Both insiders and outsiders think they are being politically 'realistic', insiders by having the ear of elected politicians, and outsiders by pointing out that this has not and will not deliver the requisite transformative social change. The second point is that one of the things missing in these reports is a theoretical appraisal of precisely what can be done and how. This lacuna is directly addressed in Chapter Eight. In the meantime, it is time to discuss aspects of the effectiveness or otherwise of systems health care delivery, starting with the NHS but extending to international comparisons.

THREE

Markets, profits and health care

Every society has had its way of dealing with impaired individual and community health, some more organised than others. While it has proved tempting to many modern Western observers to dismiss early healing systems as primitive, at least until the emergence of fully fledged agrarian states around 3000 BC, this is often to underestimate our predecessors (Graeber and Wengrow, 2021). History is in fact replete with modes of societal healing from which lessons might still be learned (see Stacey (1988) for a comprehensive but neglected sociological introduction from a feminist vantage point). Stacey defines 'health work' as embracing all those activities that involve the production and maintenance of health; the restoration of health; the care and control of birth, mating and death; and the amelioration of irreparable conditions and care of the dependent. While this is a useful reminder of the wide reach of factors that are pertinent to health and longevity and to interventions to address them, it is not necessary to explore the global trajectories of the multiple past and present forms of health work again here. Instead, I will preface an account of the emergence and travails currently facing the NHS with a few preliminary contextual remarks. The first is to approvingly note Stacey's (1988: 10) assertion that:

> Capitalism has developed from small-scale enterprise to monopoly capitalism and the associated development of international oligopolies. Contemporarily, consumer capitalism involves market control of demand, and the machinations of finance capitalists appear to render the

governments of nominally sovereign states powerless
to control their own affairs.

She goes on to insist that social structures as well as cultures change,
and understanding this is critical for explaining the evolution
of health care. Stacey's stance here is consonant with the class/
command dynamic – and by inference the GBH – though her
focus is on gender as well as class.

A second comment is on the optimal definition of a modern
'health system'. Mays (2018) suggests that the term typically refers
to all organisations, people and activities undertaken in society
in pursuit of the goals of protecting, improving or restoring the
health of a population. This includes action taken in relation to
social determinants of health. He distinguishes the health system
from the 'health care system', which is more narrowly focused on
paying for and providing health care; that is, the personal health
services oriented to meeting the health needs of individuals as
distinct from public health services oriented to population health.
Health care systems thus defined began to move away from a
reliance on markets in the liberal/early Fordist capitalism of the
late nineteenth century.

A final remark commends a framework for exploring 'local
health care systems' put forward by anthropologist Arthur
Kleinman (1985), which further contextualises what constitutes
health work in relation to personal health services. Adopting an
historical as well as an anthropological perspective, he distinguishes
between three sectors. The 'professional' sector is the one most
people think of in relation to modern Western health care: it
reflects and institutionalises an essentially biomedical approach
to classifying and responding to disease. The 'popular' sector is
the one in which most health work/care is in fact accomplished,
largely by women in the home. The acknowledgement here of the
role of 'self-care' is a reminder that only a fraction of the health
problems that people experience (that is, subjectively define as
'illness') result in a professional consultation (that is, are thereafter
'objectively' assessed in terms of 'disease'). *No modern health care
system could survive in the absence of a massive input in the guise of
largely gendered self-care.* Kleinman's folk sector refers to the myriad
alternative practitioners such as acupuncturists and osteopaths who

offer services outside of formal health care systems and whose contribution to personal health care is typically underestimated.

These three comments should be borne in mind in any assessment of the emergence and development of the NHS qua health care system, to which we now turn.

The NHS and private providers

Britain was not a pioneer of welfare or personal health care provision; on the contrary it was something of a laggard (Scambler, 2002; Scambler et al, 2014). The initial direct state involvement was a product of growing concerns about high rates of absenteeism from work and lack of fitness for war duty among working men. The result was the National Health Insurance Act of 1911. Via Approved Societies, this legislation protected part of the male population from the costs of sickness. The scheme involved contributions from the state, employers and workers and entitled beneficiaries to free primary care by an approved 'panel doctor' (that is, by an approved GP), plus a sum of money to compensate for loss of earnings. Better paid working men, women, children and older adults were excluded and had either to opt for fee-for-service primary as well as secondary care or resort to a limited and fragmentary system of 'public' (state-funded) or 'voluntary' care. The Act covered just over a quarter (27 per cent) of the population in 1911, and this had only increased to 45 per cent by the outbreak of the Second World War.

Largely middle-class pressure grew in the interwar years to extend the reach and scope of the health care services. As has been exhaustively documented, this culminated in Beveridge's (1942) blueprint against the 'five giants' of Want, Disease, Ignorance, Squalor and Idleness. His language here seems dated in the 21st century. Greener (2022) considers alternative and more contemporary nomenclatures and settles on: Inequality for Want; Preventable Mortality for Disease; Fragmenting Democracy for Ignorance; Environmental Degradation for Squalor; and Job Quality for Idleness. Beveridge's tome included plans for a national health service. Attlee's victory over Churchill in 1945 paved the way for a series of significant welfare measures, among which was the passing of the National Health Service (NHS) Act in 1946.

Introduced two years later, the NHS was explicitly founded on the principles of collectivism, comprehensiveness, universalism and equality (to which might be added that of professional autonomy). It was in some respects a compromise with the medical profession. GPs avoided what they envisaged as salaried control and became independent contractors paid capitation fees based on the number of patients on their books; the prestigious teaching hospitals were granted considerable autonomy; and GPs and, more importantly, hospital consultants won the 'right' to see patients privately. The survival of private practice was significant: 'the NHS was weakened by the fact that the nation's most wealthy and private citizens were not compelled to use it themselves and by the diluted commitment of those clinicians who provided treatment to them' (Doyal and Doyal, 1999: 364). But from this point on the state was nevertheless committed to make available primary and secondary care free at the point of service for anyone in need. These services were to be funded almost exclusively out of central taxation.

There is no need here to trace the development of the NHS in any detail since numerous comprehensive accounts can be found in the literature. But it is important to mention subsequent reforms that have a particular bearing on its precipitous decline under rentier capitalism. The recession in the 1970s caused a rethink about cost containment. In the first year of stable spending, 1950–51, the NHS had absorbed 4.1 per cent of gross domestic product (GDP). This fell steadily to 3.5 per cent by the mid-1950s, but by the mid-1960s it had regained and passed the 1950–51 level; and by the mid-1970s it had risen to 5.7 per cent of GDP. Indeed, by this time public expenditure as a whole had peaked at nearly half of GDP. Labour Prime Ministers Wilson and Callaghan took steps to rein in public expenditure, but it was Thatcher's arrival that marked a new ideology and approach. Pertinent events under and since the advent of 'Thatcherism' will be summarised here as significant 'moments' on the pathway to the disassembling of the NHS.

The first moment, the *opening broadside*, came with Thatcher's incremental challenge to the NHS and culminated in the passing of the NHS and Community Care Act in 1990. When Thatcher came to office she brought with her a set of convictions perfectly suited to the idea that welfare statism was in crisis. She capitalised on the fact that bureaucracies have long been easier to discern and condemn in the public than in the private sector (Galbraith, 1992). With a predictable agenda, Thatcher appointed Roy Griffiths from Sainsbury's to enquire into NHS management structures. The result from the mid-1980s was the termination of 'consensus management' in favour of a corporate style of management portrayed as the 'new managerialism'. In 1989, a government White Paper entitled *Working for Patients* was published and incorporated measures to promote private sector health care providers. Tax relief on private health insurance premiums for people aged over 60 years was introduced. But the main plank of the NHS and Community Care Act of 1990 was the insertion of an 'internal' or quasi-market into the NHS. This sat somewhat uncomfortably midway between a bureaucratic command and control economy and a private market. The Act pioneered 'managed competition', separating out the roles of 'purchasers' and 'providers'. Although the health service was to remain a centralised, tax-funded service accessible to all on the basis of need and (largely) free at the point of use, the barely hidden agenda was clearly to encourage the purchasing of clinical and other services from the private sector. The Act was doubtless a disappointment to many of the private sector lobbyists, notably from the USA, who had long been campaigning behind closed doors for the break-up of the NHS, but it was as far as Thatcher could go politically at that juncture (Leys and Player, 2011). NHS spending remained fairly constant through the 1980s at approximately 6.5 per cent of GDP.

The second moment was that of the private finance initiative (PFI). Introduced by John Major in 1992, this device allowed for the private sector to build and own hospitals and other health care facilities, which they then leased back to the NHS at often exorbitant rates on the back of 20–30-year deals. It suited political elites since PFI building and refurbishment did not appear on the government's books: they represented an investment of private not public monies. They were much used by the Blair and Brown New Labour governments between 1997 and 2010. As Alyson Pollock (2005) predicted, PFIs were destined to become major contributors to the indebtedness of many NHS Trusts, all the more so during the years of political austerity after 2010. As early as 1999, Richard Smith, editor of the *British Medical Journal*, denounced the PFI as 'perfidious financial idiocy' (cited by El-Gingihy, 2018). Many PFIs came with strings attached: El-Gingihy reported that by 2018 total UK PFI debt for the taxpayer was over £300 billion for infrastructure projects with a value of £54.7 billion.

The third moment might be characterised as the *coalition push*. On its election in 2010 the Cameron/Clegg government quickly backtracked on its pre-election undertaking not to engage in any further top-down reorganisations of the NHS. A mere 60 days after the election, Health Minister Andrew Lansley published a White Paper, *Liberating the NHS*, which was in fact the product of insistent private sector lobbying over an extended period. The resulting Health and Social Care Bill promised to open the door for private providers that Thatcher had left unlocked and ajar. At the core of the Bill was the proposed abolition of the extant 192 Primary Care Trusts by 2013, with GPs instead joining new 'commissioning consortia' that would control 80 per cent of the NHS budget. All NHS hospitals would become Foundation Trusts by 2014, with commissioning overseen by an NHS 'financial regulator', 'Monitor'. Health care services would thenceforth be purchased from 'any willing provider'. Doctors' professional bodies were sceptical of the Bill but fell short of outright opposition; nor did public protests prevail. The Health and Social Care Act was passed in 2012. As Leys and Player (2011) have shown, for-profit providers of services had not only lobbied the Conservatives intensively before the 2010 election but were intimately involved in the thrust and composition of the Act (via the Future Forum). Much of this lobbying was wrongly portrayed as 'internal to the NHS' rather than external lobbying.

If the 2012 Act further opened the door to private providers, a tranche of additional extra-legal 'devices' was put in place by stealth and under the public radar. Lansley's successor as Health Minister, Jeremy Hunt, already on record as personally favouring NHS privatisation (see Stone, 2016), championed a series of initiatives which, whatever merits might be claimed for them, were also designed to accelerate the privatisation of the NHS in England. This needs explicating in some detail. A new model of care through Clinical Commissioning Groups via Accountable Care Organisations (ACOs) was introduced, and on Hunt's watch a plan devised to 'bundle up' services into 'giant contracts' awarded by Clinical Commissioning Groups – and local authorities – to ACOs. ACOs comprised Multi-Speciality Community Providers (MCPs) and Primary Acute Services (PASs), which could involve private and/or public providers. ACOs could subcontract and sub-subcontract for services. And MCP and PAS providers could form Special Service Vehicles, a device to clandestinely engage the likes of private health insurers, property companies and investment bankers. A local service operating under the NHS brand could thenceforth be owned by an American private equity company without service users being any the wiser.

Consider, for example, the case of Operose. Operose was formed early in 2020 when the American company Centene Corporation combined its two existing UK subsidiaries, The Practice Group (TPC) and Simply Health. Around the same time Centene increased its stake in UK-based health care by investing in Circle Care (a 40 per cent stake according to Company House). In 2021 Operose acquired AT Medics, in the process taking over its GP contracts in London. Previously owned by six GP directors, AT Medics had been operating 49 practices across 19 London boroughs, offering services to around 370,000 people and employing 900 staff. On being acquired by Operose, its directors resigned and were replaced by Samantha Jones (CEO of Operose, ex-head of NHS England's new care models programme, former chief executive of Epsom and St Hellier University Hospitals and West Hertfordshire Hospitals Trust, and subsequently Prime Minister Boris Johnson's health adviser). A case brought by a patient at an AT Medics surgery protesting the award of dozens of contracts to Operose was dismissed by a High Court judge in February 2022.

At the time of writing, the Operose website lists contracts for 20 GP surgeries, plus a treatment centre in Birmingham and nine ophthalmology services. It also lists the contract for AT Medics to provide services for all of Croydon and part of the South-West London Clinical Assessments Service. With the addition of the 49 AT Medics contracts already mentioned, the company will have 69 surgeries and become the largest GP surgery network in the UK. A BBC Panorama investigation shown on 13 June 2022 drew on the research of an undercover reporter to conclude that Operose employs less-qualified US-style Physician Assistants (PAs) to see patients without proper supervision. Administrative staff confirmed that some correspondence had not been processed and seen by a GP or pharmacist for up to six months. Working as a receptionist at one of the surgeries the undercover reporter quoted one GP as saying that they were short of eight doctors and that the practice manager said they hired less-qualified PAs because they were cheaper than GPs. Centene/Operose, in short, are in it to make money and they and their like are permeating the NHS with the covert approval of successive governments.

The most recent of the series of top-down reorganisations of the NHS occurred in 2022 by means of the Health and Social Care Act passed into law that year. It represented a further shift towards the 'Americanisation' of the NHS, and once again it is in the detail that this is apparent. The Act established Integrated Care Systems (ICSs) as commissioners of local NHS services, while also granting the minister ultimate authority over the health service. Each ICS has two components: the Integrated Care Board (ICB) and the Integrated Care Partnership (ICP). ICBs will be responsible for the NHS functions of the ICSs, while ICPs will oversee their wider public and populations health work. What this means, in effect, is that existing Clinical Commissioning Groups will be absorbed into their local ICSs; and their commissioning powers and most of their staff will become part of the ICS body. The British Medical Association had expressed several concerns before the Act was passed, seeking assurances that there would be: appropriate clinical and patient involvement at every level of the ICSs; a default option for establishing the NHS as provider of NHS contracts to protect the NHS from costly procurement and fragmentation of services; guarantees that private providers would not exercise undue influence by sitting as members of NHS decision-making bodies; and safeguards and limitations over the minister's powers to avoid unnecessary political influence in NHS decision-making. Other critics have been blunter. One critique runs as follows. Now the old system of Clinical Commissioning Groups has been replaced by ICBs, it is up to NHS England not parliament to decide who each ICB will be responsible to.

It could be that ICBs will be able to challenge allocations and thereby, in effect, to select patients: new groups of people could be excluded from NHS care, as certain migrants currently are. Another criticism is that after years of NHS underfunding, and then COVID, the inevitable result will be further rationing, and care will become a postcode lottery. It will be harder to see a GP and the NHS could become a kitemark for private providers. For-profit companies will receive public monies to deliver procedures, and shareholders will be prioritised over reinvestment in the NHS. While it may be too soon to assess these criticisms, it is clear that the door to privatisation opened by Thatcher has been opened further by each subsequent piece of legislation (Roderick and Pollock, 2022). In January 2023 it was revealed via the Freedom of Information Act that Prime Minister Rishi Sunak had hosted a meeting with seven bosses from the UK's biggest private health companies to discuss how to tackle the growing NHS backlog of cases. These CEOs outnumbered the five NHS England attendees. No minutes were taken (openDemocracy, 2023).

Documenting the decline of the NHS

The top-down reorganisations of the NHS documented earlier, as well as being expensive in their own right, have been accompanied by general constraints placed on funding, most severely and obviously during the decade of political austerity introduced by the Cameron/Clegg coalition after 2010. Overall, the NHS experienced a decade of underfunding after 2010. Between 2009 and 2019 the NHS budgets rose on average just 1.4 per cent per annum, compared to 3.7 per cent average rises since its establishment. The more detailed data summarised here are taken from recent reports from the King's Fund (2022a) and the British Medical Association (2022, 2022a, 2022b) (see Scambler, 2023a). Funding for health services in England comes from the Department for Health and Social care's budget. Planned spending for 2022/23 was £180.2 billion, the majority of which would go to NHS England (£152.6 billion), with the remainder allocated to other national bodies for spending on other health-related functions such as public health. The Department's spending in 2020/21 and 2021/22 included funding to respond to COVID, with the result that the Department's budget grew rapidly between 2019/20 and 2021/22 before falling in 2022/23. Moreover, the NHS continues to face severe financial pressures, with Trusts across the country 'over-spending'. NHS England in 2013 said it faced a funding gap of £30 billion by the end of the decade. Despite this, the NHS was asked to find £22 billion in savings by 2020. The Nuffield Trust and King's Fund have shown that tight spending and increasing demand for services have already led to some treatments being rationed and the quality of care in some areas being diluted.

Referring to the hospital sector, and as Chapter Four will show, COVID exposed the fact that England does not have enough critical care beds. Bed shortages alongside high occupancy are unsafe for patients and staff. Data for the second quarter of 2022/23 indicate that bed occupancy levels in England have risen substantially and have passed the recommended safe threshold again. In fact, since 2010 average bed occupancy has consistently surpassed 85 per cent, the point at which safety and efficiency are at risk. Coming into the pandemic, England had an average bed occupancy of 90.2 per cent in 2019/20, though local variations in supply and demand have seen many Trusts regularly exceeding 95 per cent capacity in the winter months. Prior to COVID, the total English NHS hospital bed stock reduced by 8.3 per cent between 2010/11 and 2019/20 as the average daily total of available beds fell from 153,725 to 140,978 (in 1987/88 there were 299,000 beds). Issues around bed occupancy are compounded by discharge delays caused by pressures in social care. Social care has been neglected by successive political regimes and remains on the backburner despite multiple political promises to the contrary. The UK in general continues to have a very low total number of hospital beds relative to its population: the average number of beds per 1,000 people in both OECD and EU countries is 5, while the UK has just 2.4 (Germany has 7.8).

These general data on NHS expenditure and hospital capacity and care accessibility have implications for general practice. GP appointment bookings peaked over the winter of 2021. In terms of access, 48.1 per cent of appointments in December 2022 were booked to take place on the same day (85 per cent were booked to take place within two weeks); in terms of 'appointment mode',

68.3 per cent of appointments were booked to take place face-to-face. At the same time, a number of practices have closed and more than two in five (42 per cent) GPs are planning to work more flexibly and from home more. A long-term decline in GPs coincides with a rise in patient numbers. While there are 1,990 fewer fully qualified 'full-time-equivalent' (FTE) GPs now than there were in September 2015, each practice has on average 2,224 more patients than in 2015. The average number of patients each GP is responsible for has increased by 335 – 17 per cent – since 2015, and now stands at 2,273. Since 2017 the number of GPs working full-time hours or more in GP practice-based settings has been steadily decreasing. At the same time the number of GPs choosing to work less than full-time has been climbing, probably because doctors are moving to working patterns that allow them better to control their hours and workloads to reduce stress, ill-health and burnout. In reality, however, many part-time GPs often work additional unpaid hours just to get through the number of appointments, essential patient follow-ups and administrative work. In December 2022 there were 36,622 fully qualified GPs working in the NHS in England; in FTE terms, this equates to 27,375 fully qualified GPs. The overall number of GPs has seen little growth since 2015 while the number of GP partners has declined significantly. In a BMA survey, one in ten GPs said they planned to leave the NHS altogether after the pandemic. Government plans to reverse this problem have so far failed. What these data undeniably show is that the NHS has not been protected, and with predictable consequences. Health workers are complaining that they cannot do their jobs properly, and that there is a crisis of recruitment, including doctors, nurses, midwives and paramedics. The pace of change remains high, but it should be said that while I am writing this the Sunak government has just determined that NHS England must not, for the time being, recruit new staff (and NHS England is actively reducing its staff and has told ICSs to reduce their staff headcount). These issues, as well as pay constraints, are behind the plethora of strikes among health workers at the time of writing.

This is a narrative of decline. In a communication to the *British Medical Journal* one of the journal's oldest columnists, John Launer (2023), writes:

The NHS has sunk to being a cause for international shame. ... The BMJ is full of accounts of how bad things are in the NHS. I don't need to add to the list. But, as an older person, I want to state that I'm now afraid. I'm scared of dying in pain, dehydrated and unattended, on a trolley in a hospital corridor. I'm frightened that I'll end my days on a ward where the staff, however hard they try, won't have the time or resources to give me the care I need, either to cure me or to relieve my passing.

Characterising and explaining a declining health care system

Two interlocking stands of policy-induced change impacting on the NHS have been considered in some detail. The first testifies to an ongoing political disposition to favour private or for-profit service providers. This was initiated by Thatcher in the 1980s but has continued ever since, including during Blair and Brown's New Labour years from 1997 to 2010. It was on New Labour's watch that initiatives such as the formation of AT Medics – in 2004 – received positive encouragement. As mentioned earlier, the six founding 'doctorpreneurs' won several contracts under conditions allowing GP companies to run publicly funded GP surgeries and to employ doctors; patients did not pay fees but 'GP consortia' companies could profit from public NHS funds to run GP surgeries. Between 1979 and today, and increasingly since 2010, the political climate has allowed for a more determined and bolder assault on the founding principles of the NHS.

The second strand affords evidence of growing NHS funding constraints, with the notable exception of the New Labour years and, temporarily, fleetingly and against the Conservative grain, during the climactic years of the COVID pandemic. How to account for the interlocking of these two – privatisation and funding – strands? The short answer is that the underfunding of the NHS, one aspect of more a generalised welfare and public sector parsimony, *represents a deliberate strategy to create public dissatisfaction with what the Conservatives have always seen as a proto-socialist health care system, public dissatisfaction being a necessary (if not sufficient) condition for the viable replacement of the NHS by an Americanised or market-based model of health care delivery.* And this despite the fact that the American health care system is, by expert consent and evidence bases alike, the very worst health care delivery model to adopt.

This bias towards incorporating the private sector in health care should rightly be regarded as regressive, the thin end of an irrational and undesirable wedge. It is a classic case of (political) policy-based evidence substituting for (scientific) evidence-based policy. There is clear empirical evidence from comparative studies that privatised health care: augments costs because it requires an expanded bureaucracy that comes with contracts, billing and litigation; encourages 'cherry-picking', with the private providers focusing on the most lucrative work, such as hip and knee replacements; opens the way for fees to be introduced as services are cut and hospitals pushed into – often PFI-induced – debt, with for-profit companies presented as the cavalry on the horizon waiting to 'ride to the rescue'; prioritises cost of care over quality of care; leads to rationing, another trigger for patients to 'go private'; under cover of commercial confidentiality makes it impossible to properly scrutinise public spending via contracts with private providers that are primarily oriented to their shareholders; and promotes a fragmentation of health care services as these are refashioned according to market principles (Scambler, 2019).

One recent report, substituting 'In Place of Profit' for Bevan's title of 'In Place of Fear', refers to the 'corporate capture' of the NHS and uncompromisingly asserts that England's NHS services have been calculatingly pruned back from comprehensive, universal provision to make space for the global health care industry (SHA, 2023). Its authors argue

> that the industry's means for reaching into the healthcare market model include donations to MPs and, importantly, a revolving door between profit-making and state healthcare institutions. And that all such means must be understood within the context of the wider, policy drive against comprehensive/ universal medical care, which has reproduced key

elements of US government healthcare legislation and policy – notably Nixon's 1973 HMO Act and the US Affordable Care Act 2010 ('Obamacare'), and that these forays must be reversed as a precondition for recovering our illegitimately attacked NHS. (SHA, 2023: 3)

The steady shift towards an Americanised health care system in Britain should not be treated lightly. Health care spending in the US continues to be higher, both per person and as a share of GDP, than in other high-income countries. Yet the US is the only country that does not have universal health coverage. The US has the lowest life expectancy at birth; the highest death rates for avoidable or treatable conditions, the highest maternal and infant mortality and among the highest suicide rates; the US has the highest rate of people with multiple chronic conditions and an obesity rate nearly twice the OECD average; Americans see physicians less often than people in most other countries and have among the lowest rate of practising physicians and hospital beds per 1,000 population; and though screening rates for breast and colorectal cancer and vaccination for flu in the US are among the highest, COVID vaccination trails many nations (Commonwealth Fund, 2023).

The American business model of health care represents the very worst target of all to aim at. It accurately reflects the deep economic and social inequalities existing in that society. US health care expenditure rose 2.7 per cent in 2021, reaching $4.3 trillion or $12,916 per person. As a share of the nation's GDP, health spending accounted for no less than 18.3 per cent. This makes it the highest spending country worldwide. Germany comes next at $7,382 per head, with the UK coming in at 15th on $5,387 per head. Moreover, the American health care system is singularly deficient in that it both fails to cover all its population and leaves poorer segments of the population effectively threatened by intolerable debt or abandoned at the time of greatest need. In 2022 US health care expenditure continued to be focused significantly on private insurances (about a third), while public insurance programmes Medicare and Medicaid accounted for 24 per cent and 19 per cent, respectively. Out-of-pocket health care expenses have now exceeded $1,000, with physician and dental services and prescription drugs accounting for the largest proportion of out-of-pocket expenses for US residents (Vankar, 2022).

The situation in the UK at present is one of relentless privatisation by stealth. As Chapter Five will graphically illustrate, the advent of COVID has shone an especially harsh light on the insistent lobbying and 'purchasing' of politicians in the Westminster government by means of Conservative Party donations and the phenomenon of the 'revolving door' (namely, lucrative offers to recruit politicians to consultancies and the boards of companies when they leave office). For a sociological key to unlock this ensemble of suspect and underhand processes we can return once more to the class/command dynamic. It is this dynamic that is critical to accounting for the social structural causes of the decline of the NHS and its incremental privatisation in rentier capitalism, particularly in England, just as it is for the social structural input into the social determinants of health and the persistent and growing health divide discussed in the last chapter. But it is not of course the only social structure or set of enduring relations that matter, as will become apparent in the next chapter on aspects of our 'fractured society'.

FOUR

The structure/culture axis

Health affords an excellent lens through which to view rentier capitalism's *fractured society*. We now inhabit a society in Britain in which the super-rich have entered a stratosphere of capital and income prosperity; their close class allies – Byrne and Ruane's (2017) 'concierge class' – are being well rewarded for their services; middle-class incomes are typically being squeezed; and many working-class families are struggling to make ends meet, with some of their number falling through the increasingly parsimonious welfare safety net to indebtedness and even homelessness. This is not unique to Britain, though, as we shall see, the gap between 'top and bottom' in Britain's notably extreme form of rentier capitalism is well documented (Christophers, 2020). Social theorist Peter Engelmann (Badiou and Englemann, 2019: ix) comments in general terms on the shift that has occurred with the advent of rentier capitalism in and beyond the Occident:

> The gap between rich and the poor, both in national and international terms, is widening in grotesque fashion. ... None of the privileged groups, however, needs fear being called to account for making bad decisions or causing social damage on a scale that would match exorbitant incomes. For a long time, poverty seemed concentrated in the Third World, but now the Third World is coming to us, and the falling wages and reduced income possibilities resulting from globalisation create a fear of social decline, even in Western societies, and accelerate actual decline.

Box 4.1 provides a broad-brush characterisation of what I have analysed in detail elsewhere as our currently fractured society (Scambler, 2018). As I hope to show in this chapter, this set of compelling features of 'a fractured society in a fractured world' afford a context that extends and lends further empirical sustenance to Engels' proposition that *the health effects of capitalist exploitation can be categorised as 'social murder'* (Medvedyuk et al, 2021).

Box 4.1: Eight features of the fractured society

Environmental threat: humans have penetrated, and now reflexively shape, two historic 'givens': (i) the external or natural world, and (ii) human nature. This penetration is now established as hazardous, with predictions about global warming in particular causing widespread scientific concern. We are all of us now inhabitants of Beck's (1982) 'risk society'.

The nomadic proletariat: environmental threat is one motive for the upsurge in global migration, others being political or military conflict, absolute and relative poverty, and a desire to join family and kin. One in 110 people worldwide are currently 'displaced'. For all Beck's writing of the 'boomerang effect' of contemporary mega-risks, it is typically the global poor who remain on the front line.

The new inequality: escalated and escalating levels of material inequality are another fracturing property of financialised capitalism. According to the latest Oxfam assessment, in 2020, the world's 2,153 billionaires have more wealth than the 4.6 billion people comprising 60 per cent of the global population. A tiny fraction of the super-rich in Britain, well under 1 per cent, have seen their capital grow while the middle classes have been squeezed and stretched and the working classes have often experienced a – sometimes precipitous – decline. As for income, the top CEOs in the FTSE 100 earned the average annual salary in the first 33 hours of 2020.

Class and precarity: as the emergence of an exclusive band of super-rich alongside growing poverty testifies, class relations are biting deeper into people's lives even as the prospects of growing class consciousness seem to be diminishing. Standing (2017) is right also to note a widespread 'precarity', which captures a new cross-class insecurity around jobs, wages and prospects.

Post-national 'othering': nation states remain critical global actors, but post-national 'imaginary communities' have assumed an increasing salience, perhaps most dangerously in the wake of new patterns of migration and asylum-seeking, but extending also to the long-term sick, disabled and under- and unemployed, against whom stigma has been 'weaponised' (that is, blame appended to shame) (Scambler, 2020).

Gender dissolution: capitalism has always been gendered and racialised and relations of class have utilised and exploited this. Obstinate patriarchal relations have retained their vibrancy in financialised or rentier capitalism, a global 'feminisation of poverty' has been documented, and in Britain a cultural and rights-based challenge to cis-oriented binaries has been mounted under the rubric of a putative fourth wave of feminism. The women's movement has, as a result, become fragmented.

Cultural disorientation: there has emerged a relativisation or 'post-modernisation' of culture during financial capitalism that is functional for – though not determined by – it. As Lyotard (1984) claimed, *universal* 'grand' narratives have been displaced by *relativised* '*petit*' narratives, yielding a 'confused', pick-and-mix recipe for identity-formation as propitious for absolutes and fundamentalisms as it is antipathetic to rational positioning.

Disconnected fatalism: a step beyond disorientation is what I term 'disconnected fatalism', which denotes feelings of abandonment, bitterness, hopelessness and kindred aspects of vulnerability. It clusters among the working class, and most conspicuously among the un- and underemployed in the former mining and manufacturing communities of the Midlands and the North.

Source: Adapted from Scambler (2018, 2023)

In the opening section of this chapter, I offer a summary – a Weberian ideal type – of the nature of rentier capitalism that draws especially on the contributions of Brett Christophers. Christophers defines rent as payment for an economic actor, the rentier, who is in receipt of that rent *purely by virtue of the control exercised over something valuable*. The 'something' here is referred to as an 'asset'. Some assets are physically constructed, in virtual if not in actual space, such as housing, telecommunications, infrastructure and digital platforms; while others are purely legal, for example, intellectual property rights and outsourcing contracts; and others simply exist spontaneously, such as land and natural resources. No asset, no rent, no rentier. Rentier capitalism is a system based on 'having' not 'doing'. It is a form of 'balance-sheet capitalism'. For the likes of Smith and Ricardo, Marx too, rent was essentially 'land rent'. Now, rent remains payment for monopoly control of an asset, but the asset need not be land. If 'normal' levels of profit are those that can be made in a competitive environment, rents are the 'excess' returns afforded by any departure from that idealised scenario: rents are the abnormal profits occasioned by the capitalist power to monopolise a market. In the case of bankers, the rent can be regarded as the amount of their income that they are able to command over and above what would be required to get them to perform their activities. In sum, Christophers sees rent as *income derived from the ownership, possession or control of scarce assets under conditions of limited or no competition.* He goes on to insist that rentier capitalism not only acts to depress capitalist innovation and dynamism but is also a major mechanism for producing inequality. This lays bare its relevance: (i) for a viable sociology of health and health inequalities, and (ii) for the culpability for Engels' 'social murder' of members of that fragment of the 1 per cent that I have called the capital monopolists. Christophers (2020: 110) writes:

> Naturally, the configuration and weighting of asset portfolios and sectoral rentier forces will vary between countries ... finance and natural resources play a disproportionately significant role in the UK economy. Moreover, it is hard to imagine that any national government competes with the UK's in the extent to which it has advanced down the road of enabling contract rentiers and infrastructure rentiers through outsourcing and privatisation, respectively.

Moreover, it is not only Conservative governments in the UK that are sympathetic to the capital monopolists. In an article in the *New Statesman*, Christophers (2023a) writes:

> The striking extent to which British lives are already fashioned by asset managers made it all the more jarring

when it was reported recently that the Labour leader Keir Starmer and shadow chancellor Rachel Reeves have furtively been conducting a 'charm offensive' with senior executives at Blackstone, Brookfield and other leading industry groups.

Blackstone and Brookfield are leading asset managers. Asset managers collectively own global housing and infrastructure assets worth, at a minimum, $4 trillion.

This brief account of rentier capitalism, or as Christophers (2023) has since re-characterised it, the 'asset manager society', underpins the class/command dynamic. Strategic and self-serving decisions clandestinely taken by unaccountable capital monopolists and their allies, and subsequently translated into power/influence over politicians both in government and in opposition, and penetrating the multi-layered apparatus of the state, constitute a formidable starting point for a macro-sociology of population health and health inequalities. We are indeed run by a seemingly unassailable governing oligarchy or plutocracy. It is little wonder that social, material and health inequalities are deepening, or that well-intended recommendations for addressing them effectively are withering on the vine.

Medvedyuk and colleagues (2021) reviewed 62 papers by researchers across the globe, discerning several different social determinants of health classified under the rubric of capitalist exploitation and explicitly involving charges of social murder. The first and most prominent of these determinants was *living and working conditions* (considered in 41 of the 62 papers). While the salience of class and of versions of the class/command dynamic were apparent through these papers, race and colonialism were highlighted in a third and gendered exploitation in several others. Short (2010: 842) actually commended the concept of 'genocide' in relation to the treatment of indigenous peoples, employing the term social murder to refer to those extreme conditions of life which result in early death and disease, a 'by-product of an incompatible expansionist economic system'. A second determinant (reported in 39 papers) was *housing*. As well as addressing issues such as the generalised scarcity of decent, affordable properties, five papers concentrated on the specific phenomenon of the Grenfell Tower fire in London. Tombs (2020) interpreted the fire as a case of 'state-corporate violence' linked to the systematic dismantling of longstanding building regulations under a politics of austerity 'justified' by neoliberal ideology. Leading Labour politician John McDonnell used the term social murder to describe the tragedy at Grenfell Tower.

Unsurprisingly given the contents of numerous World Health Organization (WHO) and British reports from Black onwards, *poverty* was a third social determinant of health listed, judged a result of capitalist exploitation in 40 papers. According to the Joseph Rowntree Foundation's 'UK Poverty 2023', one in five of the UK population – 13.4 million people – were in poverty in 2020/21. Of these 7.9 million were working-age adults, 3.9 million were children and 1.7 million were pensioners. Poverty for families receiving Universal Credit or equivalents remained very high, at 46 per cent. There were strong variations by race/ethnicity, with around half of all people in households headed by someone of Bangladeshi ethnicity in poverty, and with more than 40 per cent in households headed by a person of Pakistani or Black ethnicity in poverty (more than twice the rate of people in households headed by someone of white ethnicity).

The fourth determinant was *health inequalities* (examined in 30 papers). Class, race and gender once again provide significant themes. Borras (2020: 12), who commends an intersectional approach to health inequalities and inequities, arrives at the following conclusions:

> [T]he three fundamental societal systems that underlie class-, race/ethnicity-, and gender-based health injustice are neoliberal capitalism, structural racism and patriarchy. These systems act in silos or combination to shape economic maldistribution, cultural misrecognition, and political misrepresentation that, in turn, whether in silos or combination, influence public policies impacting the social determinants of health such as labour, income, housing, food, and health care systems and services that result in health injustice.

In a paper that anticipates the depth consideration of the impact of, and lessons to be drawn from, COVID in the next chapter, Riley (2020: 1) draws on the historical studies of Engels and Virchow and the contemporary work of Marmot to analyse COVID-related deaths and their roots in social deprivation. The conclusion reached is that 'the poorest in society have died disproportionately of COVID-19, suggesting that the social murder observed by Engels in 1845 is still going on today'.

The fifth social determinant in the list constructed by Medvedyuk and colleagues is *neoliberalism*, which was mentioned in 26 papers (15 of them published post-2019). Prominent among the themes explored under this rubric is the ideological cover that neoliberal thinking provides for wide-ranging destructive policies that impact on structural unemployment, deteriorations in standards of living, ecological deterioration and socio-political instability. Garrett (2019: 196) suggests that we are witnessing the emergence of a new form of neoliberalism that uses 'communication of "messaging" strategies that aspire to disguise the continuing and true intent of the neoliberal project'. A sixth determinant is *deregulation* (11 out the 18 articles that feature it being post-2019). In the context of the UK, Tombs (2020) argues for a macro-social framework founded on the neo-liberalisation of public services. The products of deregulation understood in this way include austerity, de-democratisation and the kind of decline in social protection that led to the Grenfell Tower fire. Launchbury (2021) pursues a similar line in contending that deregulation led directly to the Grenfell Tower calamity, which is presented as the consequence of a privatised, unaccountable and deregulated housing system in the UK that prioritises private sector greed over residents' safety and qualifies as social murder.

The penultimate determinant to be considered here is *austerity* (a focus in 15 papers, 12 published after 2019). Engels' theme of social murder as a natural outcome of the social conditions of capitalism is assessed in terms of its effect on racialised, gendered and working-class populations. Grover (2019: 1) maintains that social assistance benefit cuts and increasing conditionality of welfare benefits can be understood as violent, resulting only too predictably in social murder. Violence is interpreted as 'using social-economic inequality and injustice to force the commodification of labour power, and a consequential creation of diswelfares that are known to be avoidable'. The final item on the list for summary here is *social assistance* (referenced in 19 articles, 11 after 2019). This literature hinges of welfare cuts, which are rightly regarded as indicative of social harm. Health-related sequelae are amplified in the UK by benefit sanctions and what I earlier referred to, under the nomenclature of the stigma/deviance dynamic, as the 'weaponisation of stigma', namely, an appending of blaming to shaming which can render those affected 'abject' and vulnerable to physical and mental health problems (Scambler, 2020).

I have dwelt in some detail on this summation of studies of social determinants of health that use Engels' enduring rubric of social murder because it reveals and illustrates the leading mechanisms bridging the gap between the self-serving strategic behaviours of the 'greedy bastards' of the GBH and the political elite and the maldistribution of health in the British (and other) populations, and because it rightly deploys Engels' notion of social murder in this context. I turn now to the roles played by culture and agency and how these are causally implicated in the deepening of the splits and fissures of the fractured society and, directly and indirectly, in the decline of the health care system and underwriting of health inequalities.

Cultural relativity and further macro-social dynamics

Cultural relativity bears on all eight of the characteristics of the fractured society in Box 4.1, albeit more directly on some than on others (for example, gender dissolution, cultural disorientation and disconnected fatalism). As mentioned earlier, Lyotard's (1984) *petit* narratives have displaced longstanding Western Enlightenment-oriented *grand* narratives holding up the idea of progress towards the good society. These *petit* narratives, instead, offer up multiple short-term options for consumption-led identity-formation, and in the process fuel identitarian politics. As insisted previously, it is not that identities are unimportant, rather that the significance of social structures goes missing. The net result has been a proliferation of 'culture wars', replete with ubiquitous references to 'post-truth', 'fake news', 'cancel culture', 'gaslighting', hate speech', and so on. It is as if everything is up for grabs and any antagonists are beyond the pale. I have elsewhere characterised this new phase of cultural relativity as more akin to the disinhibition occasioned by excess alcohol consumption than a genuine sign of a new emancipatory cultural thrust (Scambler, 2018). Paradoxically, it encourages rather than discourages the emergence of fundamentalisms as people long and seek for certainty in the uncomfortable midst of manifold uncertainty.

These are the symptoms of what Bauman (2007) calls our 'liquid times' (his subtitle is 'Living in an Age of Uncertainty'). While he finds positive things to say about a more generalised public acceptance of the 'messiness' of contemporary society, he is more concerned about the nature and properties of the many uncertainties that are the inevitable concomitants of this. These uncertainties, he argues, have become individualised or 'private' matters. Ritzer (2003: 243) elaborates:

> Faced with private fears, postmodern individuals are also doomed to try to escape those fears on their own. Not surprisingly, they have been drawn to communities as shelters from these fears. However, this raises the possibility of conflict between communities. Bauman worries about these hostilities and argues that we need to put a brake on them through the development of solidarity.

There is a general point to be emphasised here. Cultural relativity, manifested in the family of phenomena associated with the culture wars, is functional for the structural status quo that comprises rentier capitalism. This is because it does away with the very notion of an evidence-based and rationally compelling case for any alternative: in effect, anything goes. We have entered an era of individualised 'life politics'. I have paraphrased Bauman in these words:

> In liquid modernity the options to disavow one's individualism and to decline to participate have been removed. How one lives adds up to a biographical solution to systemic contradictions. The contradictions

67

and their associated risks remain, but the duty to confront and deal with them has become individualised and a matter of personal responsibility. Bauman argues too that a gap is opening up between individuality as fate and the capacity for self-assertion. This 'capacity', he suggests, now falls well short of what is required for genuine, 'authentic' self-assertion. (Scambler, 2018: 137)

People may feel 'subjectively' free(er) in rentier capitalism, independently of their objective circumstances; *but they have lost 'objective' freedom in that their actual capacity to act, to make a difference, has been further eroded.* This adds up to a new form of neo-conservatism. Our relativised culture, in short, allows rentier capitalism to flourish even as we inspect ourselves in the mirror.

Up to this point, two dynamics have been introduced and attributed causal powers relevant to the social maldistribution of health and longevity and the declining accessibility and efficacy of health care services, namely, the class/command and stigma/deviance dynamics. The third is the 'insider/outsider dynamic'. Rentier capitalism's cultural relativity is significant here. It has led to cultural disorientation and a sometimes despairing, sometimes desperate, drift towards fundamentalist thinking and populist engagement. The diminished salience of social structures and relations like those of class for identity-formation and a sense of self has prompted a degree of cultural disinhibition. 'Othering', or 'outsidering', has become easier. There is ample evidence in the UK and throughout much of the European Union, for example, that the insider/outsider dynamic, allied with the stigma/deviance dynamic – both involving a politics of othering – has led to a widespread recasting of refugees and asylum seekers as parasitic economic migrants. This is a social phenomenon with deep tap roots in imperialism, colonialism and racism. In this way, as we shall see in Chapter Five, on COVID, the insider/outsider dynamic has a strong ethnic or racial bias (see, for example, UK Prime Minister Theresa May's 'hostile environment' policy and the ongoing 'Windrush' scandal affecting West Indian migrant families and kin from the 1950s and 60s onwards).

The fourth dynamic is the 'party/populist dynamic'. This has to do with the class dealignment in party political voting in the UK, which is in part a by-product of the intrusion of cultural issues. But in the UK as elsewhere the formerly stable and secure mainstream political parties are being challenged by populist movements. In the words of Nancy Fraser (2019), the pre-existing 'hegemonic bloc', articulated in the form of 'progressive neoliberalism', has recently subsided into a period she describes as an interregnum. The two main candidates to replace progressive neoliberalism as hegemonic bloc, she suggests, are 'reactionary populism' and 'progressive populism'. There is more than an echo of Fraser's analysis in the UK in the late 2000s, with the Conservative Party under Prime Ministers Johnson, Truss and at the time of writing Sunak representing a racialised form of reactionary populism (much in evidence around Brexit), and the brief, but speedily terminated Labour Party flirtation with progressive populism under the leadership of Corbyn. An interregnum it may be, but in early 2023 it looks very much as if an element of neoliberal governmental stability, however precarious, has returned. I have characterised this present period as primarily one of state authoritarianism (Scambler, 2020a).

A fifth and final dynamic is the 'elite/mass dynamic'. This avers that rentier capitalism has witnessed a growing gap not only between rich and poor but also between elites across society and the mass of the population. While UK elites – and these include not only leading politicians, City of London bankers, CEOs and High Court judges, but also people such as mainstream news editors and journalists – have for a long time recruited from narrow, privileged social circles, there has grown in recent decades an extended political, social and cultural space between the movers and shakers and the moved and shaken. This has had the effect of diminishing even further the potential for either individual agency or collective or mass agency. Yet given sufficient provocation, I shall argue later, it has not altogether vanquished this potential.

Taking stock

This is a convenient juncture to take stock of the lessons of the narrative to this point, having briefly dwelt on changing historical patterns of disease and, with special reference to England and the UK, health inequalities and the deterioration in the NHS from the 1980s onwards. How especially do the general relations between structure, culture and agency, and more particularly the class/command, stigma/deviance, insider/outsider, party/populist and elite/mass dynamics, help us grasp the significance of this era of rentier capitalism for health?

First, a few more observations on structural relations of class are required and a convenient point of departure is offered by Erik Ohlin Wright (2015) in his collection of essays on social class. He distinguishes between: (i) class as individual attributes (the stratification tradition); (ii) class as opportunity hoarding (the Weberian tradition); and (iii) class as exploitation and domination (the Marxist tradition). Adjusting his own earlier unapologetically Marxist stance, he calls for what he terms 'pragmatic realism'. The individual attributes approach, in a nutshell, holds that when the different attributes of individuals and material conditions of life 'broadly cluster together', these clusters can reasonably be called classes. Wright cites Mike Savage's Great British Class Survey, which draws on Bourdieu's theories to define class in terms of three dimensions of economically relevant resources: economic capital, cultural capital and social capital (see Savage, 2015). The question of how many classes was empirically distinguished based on the ways in which indicators of these three dimensions of individual attributes cluster together. Seven classes emerged: elite, established middle class, technical middle class, new affluent workers, traditional working class, emergent service workers and precariat. For Wright what is problematic in the individual attributes approach is that it focuses on the acquisition of telling attributes for attaining economic advantaged social positions but neglects consideration of inequalities in the positions themselves.

The class as opportunity hoarding approach hinges on social closure, or the idea that if jobs bring high incomes and special advantages it is important that the incumbents of those jobs have the means at their disposal to exclude others from accessing them. Educational credentials as well as admission procedures, tuition fees and other blocks to higher education come into play. While credentialing and licensing are especially important, other devices include colour bars, marriage bars and gender exclusion, as well as religion, cultural style, manners and accents. Wright also highlights the part played by 'private property rights in the means of production' as a pivotal form of exclusion. Sociologists and others who adopt an opportunity hoarding approach tend to support a threefold categorisation of class: capitalists (as defined by private property rights in the means of production), the middle class (defined by mechanisms of exclusion over the acquisition of education and skills), and the working class (defined by their exclusion from both higher education credentials and capital). The principal difference between the individual attributes and opportunity hoarding approaches is that the economic advantages people get from being in a privileged class position are 'causally connected' to the disadvantages of people excluded from those class positions (in other words, the rich are rich *because* the poor are poor).

In explicating the class as exploitation and domination approach, Wright defines domination as the ability to 'control' the activities of others, and exploitation in terms of the acquisition of economic benefits from the labouring activity of those who are dominated. Thus, all exploitation implies some form of domination, though not all domination implies exploitation. The central class division in capitalist society is between those who own the means of production (capitalists) and those who are hired to use those means of production (workers). Capitalists within this approach both exploit and dominate. Others within this class structure get their specific character from their relationship to this basic division. Managers, for example, exercise many of the powers of domination but are also subordinate to capitalists. CEOs and top managers in corporations often develop significant ownership stakes in their corporations and therefore become more like capitalists. Highly educated professionals and some technical workers have sufficient control over knowledge and skills (an increasingly critical resource) that they can maintain considerable autonomy from domination within work and limit, or possibly neutralise, the extent to which they are exploited.

In an attempt to integrate the three different – but he suggests, complementary – approaches, Wright posits a breakdown of the class structure of the USA at the beginning of the 21st century. Box 4.2 reproduces this class breakdown on the grounds that it is salient also for the UK, with the latter experiencing sustained bouts of economic and cultural 'Americanisation' in the rentier capitalism of the Thatcher years onwards. I have stuck closely to Wright's own class characterisations.

Box 4.2: The present class structure of the USA (and the UK)

An extremely rich capitalist class and corporate managerial class, living at extraordinarily high consumption standards, with relatively weak constraints on their exercise of economic power. The US class structure is the most polarised class structure at the top among developed capitalist countries (although with the UK in hot pursuit).

An historically large and relatively stable middle class, anchored in an expansive and flexible system of higher education and technical training connected to jobs requiring credentials of various sorts, but whose security and future prosperity is now uncertain.

A working class that once was characterised by a relatively large unionised segment with a standard of living and security similar to that of the middle class, but which now largely lacks these protections.

A poor and precarious segment of the working class, characterised by low wages and relatively insecure employment, subjected to unconstrained job competition in the labour market with minimal protections by the state.

A marginalised, impoverished sector of the population, without the education and skills needed for jobs above the poverty level and living in conditions that make it extremely difficult to acquire those skills. (The US is the most polarised at the bottom among developed capitalist countries.)

Wright adds that there exists in America a pattern of interaction of race and class in which the working poor and the marginalised population are disproportionately made up of racial minorities. There is more than an echo of this interaction too in the UK, as will be made clear in the next chapter, focusing on COVID.

Source: Adapted from Wright (2015)

Interestingly, McCartney and colleagues (2019) have built on Wright's pragmatic realist conceptualisation of class in an attempt to make good the lack of theory in socio-epidemiologically skewed sociological studies of health inequalities. In the process they extend Wright's analysis to accommodate an explicit reference to early years' exposures, discrimination, health behaviours and outcomes. Recalling Bukodi and Goldthorpe's (2018) stress on the importance of 'equality of condition' mentioned in the Introduction to this volume, they argue that early exposure to class brings differential opportunities anchored in underlying power relations and legal rules and 'the social class of your ancestors'. Exposure during the 'critical period' of the early years can exercise a longstanding influence on health outcomes. They then cite Bourdieu's 'habitus' – a class-based mindset and predisposition to think and act in patterned ways – and processes of distinction which are also shaped by early years' exposures and subsequently impact on the degree to which social closure and opportunity hoarding operate for different groups. Of the strong Marxist element in Wright's perspective, they write:

> The Marxist process of conflict over production determines who is able to live off the labour of others by ownership of land, business or shares; who is able to benefit from the labour of others through managerial power; and who must work under labour discipline for a living. It can best be approximated through measures of wealth (which are a source of income/rent from the labour of others) and position in the occupational structure (professional, managerial or routine work). Which group a person belongs to within the Marxist mechanism is determined partially by the underlying power relations and legal rules, for example, concerning inheritance. (McCartney et al, 2019: 15)

Referencing the theoretical contributions of Weber on social closure, these authors once more emphasise the salience of the early years for access to the occupational structure via Bourdieu's habitus and distinction, both of which are advantageous in the processes of social closure and opportunity hoarding. Finally, they acknowledge the import of group discrimination for social closure and opportunity hoarding. But they add that discrimination can occur on the basis of biological characteristics (for example, racism) and not just attributes that are socially generated: the intersectional social processes linking class and forms of discrimination are central to this model.

This model is a welcome initiative in a literature that too often focuses on (on-the-surface) patterns and neglects (beneath-the-surface) structures, powers and mechanisms that deliver those patterns (Scambler, 2018). However, what remains largely invisible in Wright's formulation of class and its elaboration and application in the hands of McCartney and his co-authors is the pivotal premiss of the class/command dynamic. I have written of the 'capitalist executive', which bears some comparison with Wright's 'rich capitalist class/corporate managerial class', but omitted in his schema, and McCartney and associates' model is my core sub-group of the capitalist executive comprising those transnational big-hitting 'capital monopolists', super-rich nomads who display neither loyalty nor commitment to any nation state; and it is this fraction of the Occupy Movement's 1 per cent who are, in my view, critical for a credible sociological theory of health inequalities. It is they who buy power to steer social and health policy their way. And as the last two chapters have indicated, it is a power they have exercised, and are exercising, to the detriment of many of the poorer and socially ailing members of British society and of their health service.

What of the other dynamics? The stigma/deviance dynamic has afforded an enhanced opportunity for the UK's governing oligarchy or plutocracy to offload responsibility for individuals' circumstances, however dire or impoverished, onto their own often narrow shoulders. This has paved the way for anti-union legislation, low pay, job insecurity, health and welfare cuts and anti-protest measures, and for the sanctioning of any 'deviants' for their non-compliance with norms newly constituted by rentier capitalism's neoliberal ideology. The inside/outsider dynamic has performed a similar role by facilitating the blaming of particular groups of deviants for societal ills, be they 'skivers', asylum seekers or migrants or British citizens from racial/ethnic minorities. It is a dynamic that provides cover for the politics of austerity and individualism via a process of deflection, that is, by othering or scapegoating certain segments of society. The party/populist dynamic belongs within this same family. It does not just reflect a class dealignment in patterns of voting in elections but is indicative of a growing tendency in rentier capitalism, gathering momentum since 2010 and perhaps peaking with the 'Brexit referendum' in 2016, for populist politics to penetrate and even threaten established party politics. After the brief Corbyn interlude, versions of right-wing and even proto-fascist populism have been accommodated within a fragile 'conservative' return to a semblance of conventional cross-party parliamentary politics that I have dubbed state authoritarianism. The elite/mass dynamic also fits with this general picture. It points to a growing economic, social, cultural and habitus gap between many political and social elites and the bulk of the population. Aided by the ubiquitous cultural relativity, this is represented by a general detachment from and curtailment – even privatisation – of what Ray Oldenburg (1989) calls 'third places', those meeting places in civil society that allow for people to meet, exchange opinions and organise to push for social, political and policy change; and this notwithstanding the advent of virtual communication via social media, WhatsApp, and so on. In many respects the masses in our fractured society have become more distal, disoriented, disconnected, fatalist and effectively disenfranchised.

The main lesson to be learned is that recommendations for change, even if advocated and promoted in elite medical circles (for example, via the Marmot reports), will only too predictably come up against intimidating structural and cultural obstacles and that these will readily undermine any potential for effective collective action for worthwhile policy reform. In the next chapter, on the impact of the COVID pandemic, more flesh is put on the political character of the fractured society offered here. It is a narrative of an increasingly authoritarian and corrupt government executive both out of touch and eschewing any form of – even parliamentary, let alone public – accountability.

FIVE

COVID-19 and the fractured society

It might reasonably be argued that in the UK in the early part of the 21st century we are facing a 'perfect storm' in the guise of climate change, Brexit, COVID, a cost of living crisis and a relativised or post-truth culture. While it is important not to be too hasty in our judgements on live topical issues such as COVID, enough is already known to make certain conclusions incontrovertible. Moreover, it provides wholesome support not only for the class/command dynamic but for the 'greedy bastards hypothesis' (GBH). COVID revealed, if any doubt remained, just how iniquitous the fissures and cleavages in the fractured society had become. As far as health is concerned, it did so via COVID-enhanced morbidity and mortality rates for those disadvantaged by structural relations of class and race in long-deprived regions, communities and neighbourhoods. At the same time, it shone the harshest of spotlights on a decade of NHS and welfare underfunding and the resultant worsening of public access to over-stretched and understaffed NHS and welfare services. Bright (2023: 230–231) has summarised some of the relevant data. From 2009 to 2015/16 local government spending was cut by 60 per cent in real terms; and the Department for Work and Pensions' budget, which administers benefits on behalf of some of society's poorest citizens, fell by just under 60 per cent. The UK's child poverty rate soared as a result of these cuts from 15.5 per cent in 2016–17 to 19.3 per cent in 2019/20 (an increase of 24.5 per cent); and the suicide rate in England and Wales increased from 9.3 to 11 per 100,000 from 2010 to 2019. The cuts placed intolerable burdens on already overworked doctors, nurses and allied health and social workers and community and residential care workers, culminating in high rates of job stress, burnout and people leaving their jobs.

However, the pandemic illustrated just how expediently and promptly a government can detect a 'magic money tree' when a potential crisis of state legitimacy is in the offing. Unsurprisingly, it afforded ready cover too for the government's longstanding agenda of involving for-profit companies in the provision of health care services, under the rhetoric of 'meeting the COVID challenge'. It also exposed afresh a high level of political corruption via the awarding of a stream of contracts to Conservative Party donors, network allies and friends, mostly for making good the short supplies of equipment. As we shall see, this was neither 'chumocracy' nor 'cronyism' but corruption pure and simple. The sequel to the multifaceted mishandling of the COVID crisis was to be Prime Minister Rishi Sunak's political resurrection of political austerity following the implosion of the short-lived, flailing and failing Truss premiership; and this new austerity has been accompanied by widespread strikes, including but by no means confined to health workers in the guise of junior doctors, nurses and ambulance personnel. At the time of writing, the possibility of a crisis of state legitimation may be back on the agenda.

COVID came to international attention with an announcement by the Chinese government on 31 December 2019 that 'a pneumonia of unknown cause' had been detected in the neighbourhood of Wuhan. Human-to-human transmission was confirmed on 20 January 2020, and COVID arrived in Europe on 24 January. The first COVID death in the UK occurred on 6 March, the World Health Organization (WHO) declared a COVID pandemic on 11 March, and the UK announced a lockdown – 'you must stay at home' – on 23 March. The new UK's Conservative Prime Minister charged with responding was Old Etonian and Oxford University educated Boris Johnson. The governance conducted on his watch exemplifies the diagnosis of the UK in terms of a governing oligarchy or plutocracy. Investigative journalist Sam Bright (2023: 24) characterises this rule as 'a state in which political leaders are dependent on, or are heavily under the influence of, wealthy individuals who derive their growing riches from the decisions taken by their accomplices in high office'.

Delay

I have commented critically elsewhere on three aspects of the response of Johnson's government (Scambler, 2020a). The first of these focuses on *delay*. For a start, and despite repeated warnings about a lack of preparedness for a pandemic, no precautionary action had been taken. In their forensic analysis of this neglect, Arbuthnott and Calvert (2021) conclude that emergency stockpiles of PPE had severely dwindled and were out of date because they had become a low priority in the years of austerity cuts. Furthermore, and even allowing for the existence of conflicting expert as well as lay opinion, there is something of a consensus among epidemiologists that the government was slow to act when the extent of the COVID threat became clear. Helen Ward (2020), an infectious disease epidemiologist, reports being worried in mid-February of 2020. In April she wrote:

> Two months on, that anxiety has not gone, although it has been joined by a sense of sadness. It's now clear that so many people have died, and so many more are desperately ill, simply because our politicians refused to listen to and act on advice. Scientists like us said lock down earlier; we said test, trace, and isolate. But they decided they knew better.

The government went on to resist mounting expert public health and public pressure for 'circuit-breaking' two- or three-week lockdowns to stall incremental waves of COVID until compelled to act, most notably in the period following the easing of restrictions over Christmas, 2020.

Strategy

My second criticism of the government's response focuses on *strategy*. While it should be acknowledged that any government would have been confronted by very real difficulties formulating a pragmatic and effective, science-based strategy to tackle a virulent infection like COVID, it rapidly became clear that the strategy Ward and numerous other leading epidemiologists recommended, in line with WHO advice, was not adopted in the UK (Horton, 2020). The government opted instead, and clandestinely, for a policy of 'herd immunity', namely, letting the virus work its way through a substantial proportion of the population to generate widespread immunity. Some interpreted this as a form of 'Social Darwinism' or the survival of the fittest. It seemed to critics that the government was open to sacrificing vulnerable segments of the population – especially the long-term sick and disabled and the elderly – as collateral damage. The government quickly denied ownership of such a policy, though suspicions that its ministers were dissembling have never gone away. The discharge of COVID patients from hospitals and into care homes and the rapid accumulation of COVID-related deaths in care homes, hospitals and in the community added further fuel to the fire. Richard Horton (2020, 2020a), editor-in-chief of the *Lancet*, described the government's response to COVID as 'the biggest science policy failure in a generation'.

Bare statistics do not reflect the amount of human suffering involved, and to this end I am including, with permission, an exchange of texts between the manager of a care home and a friend. The names of the manager and the care home have been changed in the interests of anonymity. The care home was located in the South-East of England, the area worst hit by care home fatalities. 'Lodge House' was the first care home to be opened in the locality to care for people discharged from long-term hospital care for mental health problems to facilitate a transition to living in the community. It is registered as a 'nursing care home' and is sanctioned to care for up to 55 adults, under or over the age of 65, with a special focus on dementia services. Lodge House is managed by a nurse/manager whom I will call 'Cathy'. Cathy has given her permission to access the exchange of texts sent to a friend over the period when Lodge House was riven by COVID and spontaneous and improvised managerial decision-making became the new norm.

Cathy's narrative actually begins with an account of an attack on her by a resident. It was a serious assault and she suffered psychological trauma as well as physical injury. On 29 March 2020, she wrote to a friend:

> Well, I'm still taking an assortment of tablets, plus morphine. We have no way of testing our patients at present but hopefully we will remain clear (of COVID). We are simply going from home to work and back. I am working around 6–8 hours a day and then some work at home.

In an update on 31 March, she added: 'We're down to six support staff with so many off sick. ... Food okay, but we're still waiting for government supply of masks.'

Cathy's friend noted that supplies of PPE were being diverted from care homes to hospitals in many parts of the country, to which Cathy replied:

> Yes, and that is why care homes will not accept patients from hospital, as the PPE is not sufficient protection from the virus. ... I am the only trained nurse this morning and we have fifty patients and six support partners so it's hard in the first place and I am hoping to avoid an infectious admission. ... I now have cellulitis on my face near to my eyes and nose! My GP says she has to knock me sideways with antibiotics, and if no better today I have to talk with her again. It's uphill all the way.

Later that same day Cathy explained that she had a deputy she was mentoring but that the situation was far from ideal. Although this deputy might do a shift 'in a real difficulty', her previous stints had caused considerable friction with the other staff ('she will manage the care well, but there are so many other parts to this job').

On 2 April Cathy had awful news: 'Our nursing home is owned by a married couple who are our best friends. We have just heard the dreadful news that "X" has died in (the local) hospital last night from the coronavirus. Devastated!'

Cathy was asked if she was okay, and she replied on 6 April:

I think so. Unfortunately, we may have the coronavirus in the Home. I spoke to the doctor in Public Health England as we have several patients with high temperatures. They can't arrange tests until Wednesday at the earliest [six days later]. They are currently overwhelmed. Even then only five will be tested – and no staff testing. Of course relatives are distraught. We are all wearing PPEs, but the masks will not last long. The CQC say it's hard to get anything. Quite scary but I have to reassure the staff.

A day later she wrote that: 'Today was hell. Spent hours trying to obtain masks. Some hope in the end. Some patients very sick. We are so busy.'

Then, on 9 April she updated her friend:

We heard today that the six swabs tested positive for coronavirus. We have 28 symptomatic patients. We just hope we can get through. We are all shattered. With the approval of the infection control nurse I am now instructing staff to take off all PPEs and go outside for five minutes for air. Otherwise, we are feeling faint and breathless and hot. I have a lot of staff off sick and it's a juggling act to keep the rota going successfully.

And in a second text that same day she added: 'Also I was told it's now mandatory to register with a national account our vacancies. However I will not let them force us to admit more COVID-19 patients.'

On 14 April Cathy wrote: 'I really don't know what to say or even what to expect. Now we have a donated caravan in the car park. I am ill with a temperature BUT I have to be the night sister who has gone off sick. ... The best I can offer is to be on call if they need me.'

On 19 April her health had deteriorated further:

Sorry to say I am very ill. All the people I nursed have died. I've managed to speak with one London doctor. He thinks there is just one antibiotic that may be useful. I am having diarrhoea and vomiting up to fifty times a day for five days now. [Cathy's husband] is out trying to get the script, which has proved incredibly difficult as a local GP has to agree. My employer has pulled every string possible and we think it is now solved. I am now very weak and feeling very anxious.

And on the following day, still initially with no medicine:

We are waiting to hear from the London doctor. Just hope to get the medicine today after so many abortive attempts. I still have diarrhoea and vomiting and high temperatures. ... Medicines finally arrived at midday. Evidence for effectiveness is slight but I need to try as I'm not making much progress.

There was a hint of improvement by 21 April: 'Still very symptomatic but I think there is a small improvement. I'm fighting with all my might.' And on 24 April, Cathy was able to write: 'Yes, things are getting a bit better, but it's slow. I complete the medicine today so the hope is that after this things might settle down. I am so weak after nine days of this hell.'

On 28 April: 'Just started to eat a few teaspoons yesterday. Very weak but that will pass. ... It's going to take a while.'

Progress continued to be slow, if steady, and Cathy's update on 3 May was as follows: 'I will not be going back for some time. We have only 33 patients left out of 50. There will be so much work when the Home re-opens. I am planning to do the necessary care plans from our own home. Frankly I'm terrified of returning in case of catching anything.'

On 13 May, Cathy reported on a CQC inspection of Lodge House:

I went to work for one hour as we had a CQC inspection. We did well. Anyway we now have only 34 residents, with 15 coronavirus deaths and three more who look as if they soon will die. We cannot take admissions as there are still residents with raised temperatures. I made a huge fuss with the CQC inspector about the lack of PPE from (the local council). We are now even sourcing from Germany at a huge cost. The inspector says the government gave money to [the local council] at the weekend and we can apply for a grant to help with PPE. I said it was partly the poor PPE that led to my illness. Also I requested 80 tests before I went off sick. We have emails you can see to prove that they have not arrived. The inspector is to make enquiries for us. So after six positive tests no one has felt it needful to test other residents or staff. You can imagine how relatives and staff feel!

A little later, on 17 May, Cathy was in a reflective mood:

Just wondering if there is any evidence that generally there is a misunderstanding about the skills of staff in nursing homes? I feel that when those in authority speak of carers as low skilled workers this is indicative of ignorance. I feel that this could have led to wrong decisions: in our Home we have skills that are often not present in hospital for care of the elderly. In all commentaries I've only heard one GP acknowledge this. If our work is not valued or understood, the information passed to government is bound to be at best inaccurate and would lead to disastrous decisions.

She followed this text up with another shortly after:

We now think that possibly our Home became infected when a patient who stayed in [two local hospitals] for an amputation was returned to us without testing. He was symptomatic of coronavirus and was diabetic. I do not think the hospital or ourselves recognised the significance of the diarrhoea he returned with.

On the following day, 18 May, came the final text I shall cite here: 'Well, after eight weeks the tests are arriving for residents and staff, and of course me! The army are collecting them tomorrow. This has taken eight weeks!'

This exchange speaks for itself, and with a poignant articulacy. It is not only consonant with the analysis that preceded it, it affords a blow-by-blow insider account of the side-effects of a calamitous failure of politics, policy and practice. More than this, it bears testimony to a sense of fatigue, fear, hopelessness and suffering common across many care homes in the country. Its spontaneity lends it a special intimacy.

Efficiency and effectiveness

My third critical comment concerned *efficiency and effectiveness*. The government's organisational laxity is beyond dispute. And disturbing reasons for this are emerging in ever-increasing detail. Not only did the lessons of two dry runs for pandemic preparation (in 2016 and 2019) go unlearned, but in line with the Conservative regime's opting for a bout of austerity post-2010, the NHS lost funding, the privatisation of services was encouraged, there were severe staffing cuts, formal social care was all but abandoned, stockpiles of PPE diminished, and central and local government monies committed to public health were slashed.

To this trio of critical comments might be added a fourth, *trust* (Scambler et al, in press). It is axiomatic that a high level of public trust is a precondition for the effective countering of a pandemic. The Johnson administration squandered the sympathy, understanding and, a by-product, the 'compliance' of strands of the population. This should not have occasioned surprise. Johnson is a product of 'Bullingdon Club Britain', a label referring to an exclusive Oxford University club whose carefully selected Eton and Harrow educated members oozed privilege and stood for the irresponsible, arrogant and amoral pursuit of self-interest. Bright, himself briefly a member of the Bullingdon Club but now an investigative journalist, offers a devastating judgement:

> [T]heir ineptitude cloaked by bluster and lies continues to inflict daily damage on Britain's reputation and its economic prospects. The Bullingdon generation of politicians … left no permanent monuments to their

vaulting ambition. They lied to gain power and money and had no clue what to do with either. History is unlikely to be kind to them. (Bright, 2023: 13)

Johnson, more so than fellow ex-Bullingdon Club member and British Prime Minister David Cameron before him (who left Brexit as his 'monument'), epitomises Bright's characterisation. The loss of trust under Johnson was not merely a function of inexcusable delays, a flawed strategy and inefficiency and ineffectiveness, it was compounded by government rhetoric. People were not slow to notice a yawning gap between promises and delivery. Test and trace, for example, was heralded as 'world class' even as it conspicuously faltered. Health Minister Matt Hancock used any media opportunity to talk up rather than ramp up 'test and trace', even disguising the facts that the numbers he released included test kits posted and not used/returned and that many swabs were unreliable and would need retesting. Nor were the commercial labs used to run tests sharing data with local public health groups or councils. Trust in government statements and advice around lockdowns was further eroded by examples of elite non-compliance with the rules laid down for the citizenry. Johnson's adviser Dominic Cummings' rule-breaking trip to Barnard Castle was a key incident; and this was to be followed by a series of illicit gatherings or parties in and around 10 Downing Street that became known as 'Partygate' and signalled the beginning of the end of Johnson's premiership. In early summer 2023 news of yet further Johnson parties are emerging. As we shall see later, these flaws in the Johnson government's response to COVID were to lead to many excess COVID-related deaths and might in their own right be regarded as a form of social murder. But there was another dimension to governmental policy-formation that requires commentary.

Not 'chumocracy' or 'cronyism', but corruption

Not enamoured with parliamentary procedure at the best of times, COVID provided an opportunity for the ruling Conservative Party under Johnson to sidestep accountability in the House of Commons via the expedient of emergency powers, thereby opening the door to executive decision-making: it was immediately clear that this allowed for an onus on the private or for-profit provision of services. In March of 2020 the Treasury agreed a deal to block-book the entire capacity of all 7,956 beds in England's 187 private hospitals along with their almost 20,000 staff to help supplement the NHS's efforts to cope with the unfolding pandemic. The cost of this is estimated at £400 million per month. However, the Centre for Health and the Public Interest (2021) calculates that on 39 per cent of the days between March 2020 and March 2021, private hospitals treated no COVID patients at all, and on a further 20 per cent of days they cared for only one person. Overall, they provided only 3,000 of the 3.6 million COVID bed days in this period (0.08 per cent of the total). The report's author writes: 'Despite the fact that the taxpayer paid undisclosed billions to the private hospital sector, which prevented some of the companies going bust, the official data shows that they barely treated any COVID patients and delivered less elective work for the NHS than they did prior to the pandemic.'

Secrecy around the contracts was to be maintained by ministers, NHS England and the Treasury. The Chair of the House of Commons Public Accounts Committee, Meg Hillier, went on to complain too that many millions of pounds had been spent on unfit PPE languishing in costly storage and that £530 million had been spent on the *unused* Nightingale hospitals (see Campbell, 2021).

The Conservative agenda favouring private sector health provision was addressed in Chapter Three, and that COVID should afford an opportunity for advancing this agenda by executive stealth should be no surprise. Tony O'Sullivan, a retired consultant paediatrician and co-chair of 'Keep our NHS Public' has said: 'The private sector was bailed out during Covid, has a lucrative four-year £10 billion deal ongoing and is also in a position to earn massive profits from patients forced to go privately to avoid NHS queues of 7.2 million' (openDemocracy, 2023).

But of even more concern was the blatant favouring of Conservative MPs, donors and members with VIP contracts to – allegedly – meet the challenges of COVID. In fact, COVID opened the door to a veritable gold rush for government contracts. A cross-party group of MPs castigated the government for hiding details of hundreds of COVID PPE contracts valued at more than £5 billion. But it was the test and trace system that generated the most attention. In May of 2020 Hancock appointed Dido Harding to head the NHS Test and Trace, established to track and help prevent the spread of COVID in England. The background and context of this appointment has been appraised elsewhere and is briefly summarised in Box 5.1 (see Scambler et al, in press).

Box 5.1: The rise and rise of Dido Harding & Co

Dido Harding is the daughter of John Charles Harding, 2nd Baron Harding of Petherton (and granddaughter of the 1st Baron, Field Marshall John Harding). She was educated at an independent Catholic school and Oxford University.

She joined the management consultancy firm of McKinsey & Co in 1988, prior to holding executive posts with Thomas Cook, Manpower, Kingfisher and Woolworths, Tesco and Sainsburys. She became the first CEO of TalkTalk in 2010 but was criticised when TalkTalk suffered a sustained cyberattack in 2015. The attack cost the company £60 million and 95,000 customers and she stood down as CEO in 2017.

In 2018, Harding joined the main board of the Jockey Club, which runs multiple events, including the Cheltenham Festival. Public health experts were dismayed when this 'super-spreader event' went ahead and 250,000 people packed the terraces. Matt Hancock, interestingly, is the MP for Newmarket, where the Jockey Club has major structural investments. It has been estimated that Hancock has received £350,000 in donations from wealthy people in the horseracing business. Before the 2019 election he announced: "I'll always support the wonderful sport of horse racing." The Jockey Club's premier event remains the Randox Health Grand National, and one of the government's most controversial contracts is with Randox. The global health care firm was given a £133 million deal, without advertisement or competition, to supply testing kits. Randox paid ex-Conservative MP and active 'lobbyist' Owen Patterson £100,000 per annum for 200 hours of work. Randox's testing kits were subsequently withdrawn on the grounds that they might be unsafe (Monbiot, 2020).

In 1995 Harding married John Penrose, who was elected Conservative MP for Weston-super-Mare in 2005 and held junior governmental posts from 2010 to 2019. Penrose sat on the advisory board of the right-wing think tank '1828', which campaigns for the NHS to be replaced by an insurance system (and called for Public Health England to be scrapped). He also headed the Conservative Party's anticorruption team. Dido Harding was made a Conservative Life Peer in 2014.

When Harding was appointed head of NHS Test and Trace, the membership of her team was kept secret. It has since been leaked. It included only one public health expert but found space for a former executive from Jaguar Land Rover, a senior manager from Travelex and an executive from Waitrose. Harding's adviser was Alex Birtles, who worked at TalkTalk with her. Subsequently, Mike Coupe, an executive at another of her old firms, Sainsburys, was also appointed (Monbiot, 2020).

Source: Adapted from Scambler et al (in press)

'NHS Test and Trace' was always something of a misnomer since, as is apparent from Box 5.1, its orientation from the very start was towards the private sector. It was to provide a rich seam of profits. A contract officially priced at up to £410 million was handed out to Serco. It appears that this contract contained no penalty clause, meaning that even if Serco were to fail to satisfy its terms it would be paid in full. In the event, Serco subcontracted contact tracing jobs to another company. Serco's CEO was Rupert Soames, whose partner is a Conservative donor and whose brother is ex-Conservative MP Nicholas Soames. Junior Conservative Health Minister Edward Argar is a former lobbyist for Serco. In March of 2021 it was reported that Rupert Soames had been paid £4.9 million for 2020 (Jolly, 2021).

Although official figures have remained hard to come by, the final bill for private sector contracts will amount to several billion pounds. Additional contracts for managing the procurement of ventilators and PPE, and extending to the monitoring of contracts, were awarded to management consultants and amounted to hundreds of millions of pounds. The coordination of testing conducted by private sector staff was overseen by consultants from Deloitte at an undisclosed cost. Junior Deloitte staff supplied to another public body, the British Business Bank, which coordinated COVID financial support packages, reportedly cost taxpayers salaries comparable to that of the prime minister. Nor have these extravagant costs been accompanied by efficiency. Handing the central tracing service to 25,000 people with no experience and only rudimentary training led to the standardisation and computerisation ('McDonaldisation') of processes to the point of blinkered ineffectiveness. It was soon apparent that the tracing of contacts of people testing positive was far lower in the central service than it was in the smaller number of more complex cases handled by local public health teams.

With the advantage of hindsight, Bright (2023: 56) pulls no punches in his interpretation of Conservative rule through the pandemic years:

> Seeing an opportunity to profit from Johnson's moral deficit – combined with the commercial opportunities provided by the pandemic – various corporate interests circled the Conservative Party. During this period, the governing party therefore acted more like a social club for the rich – a frat house for corporate interests – than a democratic body.

Jolyon Maugham (2023: 232), founder of the Good Law Project, which is (still) seeking to hold the government properly to account for its COVID-related actions, is no less damning:

> It was a looting of public resources on a grand scale. ... None of this was opportunism. The process involved ushering suppliers overwhelmingly handpicked by ministers through what was brazenly described as a VIP lane, with its own special processes and discrete team of handlers. But only suppliers lucky enough to enjoy political connections to the Conservative Party. Of the many referrals into the VIP lane from politicians, all were from Conservative MPs or peers.

The point also needs to be made that several outspoken right-wing neoliberal think tanks, housed in Tufton Street in Westminster and given plenty of airtime by the mainstream media, afforded ready ideological cover for the Conservative economic and health policies (policies sold via 'booming memes'). And to these 'influencers' must be added the bulk of the Conservative-supporting British press. The *Daily Mail* is owned through trusts based in Jersey and the Bahamas, its proprietor the billionaire Lord Rothermere. The *Daily Telegraph* is owned by Sir Frederick Barclay, who lives on Brecqou, a private island in the Channel Islands. Rupert Murdoch, worth an estimated $19 billion, controls *The Sun*, *The Times*, talkRadio, Talk TV and the publisher HarperCollins. To redeploy my earlier technical term, politically motivated 'greedy bastards' were and remain to the fore. It is worth noting too that fully a third of the mainstream media's current columnists were educated at independent schools and Oxbridge. So, the coming of COVID revealed the workings of the class-based and mass media promoted power elite of the British state – our governing oligarchy or plutocracy – in raw detail. Not chumism, not cronyism, but corruption. Reporting on their ongoing study of 'how Britain's Covid support for big business entrenched inequality', covering executive pay, shareholder dividends and wage gaps in firms that received public cash, Fooks et al (2023) conclude that their data strongly suggest that billions of pounds of public money has effectively been spent to prop up an economic model that is progressively entrenching wealth and income inequalities.

COVID and the fractured society

In likening COVID to a naturally occurring rather than artificially constructed or experimental 'breaching experiment', I have been concerned to show not just that political corruption is rife, but that the fractures in contemporary British society are deep and enduring (Scambler, 2020a). Research has shown that the years of austerity after 2010 hit the most deprived groups hardest. The measures that the Conservative governments took reduced social spending and increased taxation. Simon Williams and Martin McKee (2023) show that these austerity policies weakened the UK, allowing COVID to do more damage than it otherwise might have done. The spending gap attributed to austerity – reductions in health and social care expenditure – was 13.64 per cent between

2010 and 2015, which it is estimated led to 33,888 extra deaths in the same period. By the mid-2010s, life expectancy at older ages had begun to decline. Austerity, they argue, acts at every point on the pathways that lead to disease and premature death. They end their grim narrative of the fractured society with a warning. The COVID pandemic will not be the last. One of the optimum things we can do to prepare for future pandemics is to avoid a return to austerity.

David Stuckler and colleagues (2017) examined the evidence for austerity's impact on health in the UK and Europe through two principal mechanisms: a 'social risk effect' of increased unemployment, poverty, homelessness and other socio-economic factors (indirect), and a 'healthcare effect' through cuts to health care services as well as reductions in health coverage and restricting access to care. Their conclusions are predictable. Austerity impacted most severely on those already vulnerable, such as those with precarious employment or housing or with existing health problems. The authors emphasise that the wealthy emerged almost unscathed, while 'those without power face a future that is more precarious than ever', exacerbated by erosion of previous social safety nets. Using the concept of asset flows conducive to health introduced earlier, austerity further weakened the flows of those already experiencing a cluster of weak flows. According to a study by Walsh and colleagues (2022), and at a conservative estimate, the years between 2012 and 2019 saw approximately 335,000 additional deaths.

So the slope was significantly downward prior to the arrival of COVID on Britain's shores. Michael Marmot and colleagues (2020), at the Institute of Health Equity, have built on this bank of research to track the impact of the pandemic. They conclude that:

> The UK has fared badly. Not only does England vie with Spain for the dubious distinction of having the highest excess mortality rate from COVID-19 in Europe, but the economic hit is among the most damaging in Europe too. The mismanagement during the pandemic, and the unequal way the pandemic has struck, is of a piece with what happened in England in the decade from 2010.

Addressing the issue of the UK's 'mismanagement' directly, these authors lay stress on four points. First, both before and during the pandemic the governance and political culture mitigated against social cohesion and inclusiveness, undermined trust, de-emphasised the importance of the common good, and failed to take the political decisions that would have put the health and wellbeing of the population to the forefront. Second, the widening inequities of power, money and resources between individuals, communities and regions have generated inequalities in the conditions of life, which in their turn generate inequalities in health generally, and COVID specifically. They add that all this augurs badly for populations' health post-COVID. Third, the post-2010 politics of austerity reduced public expenditure, involving regressive cuts in spending by local government, including social care, a failure for health care spending to rise in line with demographic and historical trends, and cuts in public health spending. These cuts were in addition to cuts in welfare to families with children, in education spending per school student, and the closure of Children's Centres. England entered the pandemic years with its public services in a depleted state and its tax and benefit system disadvantaging lower income groups. And fourth, not only had population health stopped improving but there was a high prevalence of the health conditions that increase the fatality ratios of COVID. The lessons, Marmot and colleagues insist, must be learned. And they pose a key question for this volume, namely, *what sort of society do we want to build?*

It will be apparent that underlying social structures, of class in particular, plus the emergence of cultural relativity and 'culture wars', are core beneath-the-surface mechanisms. COVID put the fractures of UK society, rent by rentier capitalism, on display. But patriarchal structures are on display too once one sees through a plethora of culture wars calculated, funded and fuelled to confuse and divide (Bright, 2023). If it is not apparent from the data that women's COVID-related mortality rates exceed men's, what is beyond dispute is the enhanced 'duties of care' that have fallen to women, both as carers themselves (a critical part of Kleinman's (1985) popular sector in any local as well as national health care system) and as care workers in homes and in the community. It is a duty significantly enhanced not only by COVID and successive lockdowns, but by the growing inaccessibility of local statutory social care and of private sector social care for adults (King's Fund, 2021). Moreover, the corporate takeover plus higher rates of outsourcing of children's care have meant more children moving between short-term, unstable placements far away from their families (Wall, 2023).

As intersectional writers would rightly insist, racial structures also need to be considered in the context of COVID. In part, race 'masks' class, but the statistics on race and COVID-related morbidity and mortality require further comment. In April of 2020, a study of hospital admissions afforded the first substantive evidence that death rates were higher among black and Asian patients who had contracted COVID (see Platt, 2021). Subsequent research showed that deaths in care homes followed this same pattern. Why was this? Several factors were relevant: a greater likelihood of working in health and social care key worker occupations (notably black Africans); greater chances of having a health condition that made them especially vulnerable to COVID (notably Bangladeshis); and greater chances of living with others or in more densely occupied or overcrowded areas. But these factors did not wholly account for the racial differences, racism being another complicating factor. A study commissioned by the National Police Chiefs' Council – but not published by them – found that black people were three times more likely than white people to receive COVID fines in England and Wales (fines were also seven times more likely to be handed out in the poorest areas than in the richest) (Dodd, 2023). A comparative statistical study of race and ethnicity and COVID in the USA and the UK backed up the general findings reported here (Chun-Han, 2021). A more recent UK study of the impact of COVID on people of Black, Asian and minority ethnic backgrounds (BAME) found that BAME children experienced increased anxiety over parental employment and income; cramped housing, the absence of free school meals and a lack of access to Internet and digital services had a negative impact on their ability to stay engaged with their education during lockdown; BAME children experienced inconsistencies in policing of lockdown rules and similar inconsistencies in supporting education and mental health; BAME families were affected by low pay, precarious jobs, poor housing conditions and immigration control; BAME parents were not able to access financial support available to other workers during the pandemic; and multigenerational homes made social distancing a challenge especially in overcrowded housing (for a summary, see UCL News, 2023). For all that I have argued in this volume that class is *the* paramount social structure in capitalism and differs in this respect from both gender and race, it is clear that a broadly intersectional approach is necessary to *fully* understand and explain population health and health inequalities.

If anyone was sceptical about the UK's enduring class structure and companion divisions of gender and race, COVID has provided further corroboration, as it indeed has for the class/command dynamic. The class/command dynamic and the GBH are, in my view, fully consonant with the now vast body of national and international sociological and socio-epidemiological research on population health and health inequalities. Bambra and colleagues (2021: 28) draw on the notion of a 'syndemic' to capture COVID's differential impact:

> A syndemic exists when risk factors or comorbidities are intertwined, interactive and cumulative, adversely exacerbating the disease burden and additively increasing its negative effects. ... We argue that for the most disadvantaged communities, COVID-19 is experienced as a syndemic: a co-occurring, synergistic pandemic which interacts with and exacerbates their existing chronic health and social conditions.

This has obvious ramifications for attempts to address the issue of appropriate and *effective* health and health care reforms, and for understanding and explaining why the society-wide reforms commended by Michael Marmot and others have not, and cannot, be implemented. The deep and abiding structural obstacles are too great. To date, too few scholars and reformers have been willing to front up to this uncomfortable truth.

But there is another dimension to this quandary. It is a major contention of this volume that the health of populations in particular nation states such as the UK can no longer, if they ever could, be considered in isolation from global health. This is not just a 'moral' issue about the extent to which any increase in the 'effectiveness' of British reforms might be at the price of increases in the rates of exploitation of other countries and the resultant diminution of population health and health inequality in those countries. We have now entered a phase of rentier capitalism in which it has become progressively and more urgently apparent that Beck's (1982) risk society is here to stay. The age of the Anthropocene is upon us. Chapter Six begins the challenging task of unravelling what this might mean not only for us as British citizens but for contemporary sociologists of health and health care systems. Ironically, even as more emphasis globally as well as in Britain is being placed on preventive health care, espousing the benefits of regular (DIY) health testing – alongside genetic mapping – to uncover diseases before they become serious (and expensive), we are moving, globally and nationally, in the opposite direction, intervening, *if at all*, only after people have been pushed into unemployment and relative and even absolute poverty (Bright, 2023).

SIX

The challenge of global inequality in the Anthropocene

We have become more reflexively aware that we now inhabit a 'world risk society'. In 1999, Beck defined this in terms of an accumulation of risks – ecological, financial, military, terrorist, biochemical and informational – that have coalesced into an overwhelming presence in our contemporary world. Beck's risks remain real and intimidatory, but it is perhaps the notion of the Anthropocene that has concentrated the minds of scholars across several disciplines into the 21st century and underlined the threat of genuinely globalised hazards. The Anthropocene will be analysed in Chapter Seven, but it will be helpful to define it briefly here because there is a sense in which its impact via climate change has come to symbolise the vital interlinking and interdependence of the populations of a world 'artificially' segregated by nation state. Its implications for the human species per se will be considered in the next chapter. All that is required at this point is an abbreviated definition of the Anthropocene. In a paper published in *Nature* in 2015, Lewis and Maslin cite evidence that the Earth may have entered a new human-dominated geological epoch, the Anthropocene, succeeding that of the Holocene. They consider how best to date the advent of this epoch and highlight two trigger dates, 1610 and 1964. The year 1610, in the 'long sixteenth century' during which capitalism took hold (see Box 1.1), was selected because it allegedly marked the beginning of the 'age of man': it was when Europeans in the Americas prompted a transition that was to become an unprecedented impact on the planet. It has also been suggested that this was around the time that the low point of atmospheric carbon dioxide (CO_2) concentrations was registered (as recorded in ice cores). This, it is hypothesised, likely occurred because of a drastic reduction in farming in the Americas, representing what was to prove an irreversible transfer of crops and species between the new and old worlds. The year 1964 was considered because it witnessed a peak in radioactive fallout following nuclear weapons testing prior to the test ban treaty coming into effect. It is not necessary either to adjudicate or even to analyse these still-controversial claims now (see Chapter Seven). The point to signal now is that as the discussion in the present chapter turns to global health issues it should be borne in mind that what is now often accepted as the Anthropocene is upon us. If the central thesis of this chapter is that it is no longer either satisfactory or acceptable to consider health and health care in England and Britain while neglecting the global context, the central theme of the next chapter will be that the character of the Anthropocene demands that we totally rethink what constitutes a healthy population, or a 'healthy society', as the future impinges on the present in the guise of a threat.

Box 1.2 showed the very different leading causes of death in low-income countries when compared to medium- to high-income countries. This is consistent with long recognised propositions that material standards of living matter for health, as do levels of equality. It is clearly not possible to sample a heterogeneous range of individual societies and cultures in the space available here. It is important for the argument in this chapter, however, to begin by gaining some understanding of the extent of current levels of inequality between as well as within (developed Western) nations. The World Bank recently released a revised set of poverty and inequality data. This set used updated methods and included an adjustment to the International Poverty Line (IPL) deployed to measure extreme poverty (see Roser, 2021). The IPL was reset from $1.90 to $2.15 per day. These astonishing figures testify to the fact that a huge majority of the world is *very* poor, with the poorer half of the world, nearly four billion people, living on less than $6.70 per day. If a person is living on $30 a day, he or she belongs within the richest 15 per cent of the world's citizenry ($30 a day corresponds approximately to the poverty lines set in high-income countries). We have already noted that inequality within societies can be high: it is high and has got higher in the UK for example, though the USA is the high-income country with the most glaringly high rate of inequality. But much of global inequality is inequality between countries. This means vast inequalities in living conditions. Indeed, because a reasonable income is a basic precondition for good living conditions, many other inequalities are found to map onto economic inequality.

It was noted earlier in this text that life expectancy in the poorest countries is around 30 years shorter than in the richest countries. As an abundance of comparative research has shown, where incomes are higher people live longer; children and mothers die less often; doctors and health workers can focus on fewer patients; people have better access to clean drinking water and electricity; they have more free time and can travel more; they have better access to education and better learning outcomes; and people say they are more satisfied with their lives. Reflecting on the World Bank data, Roser invites his readers to ponder a world without any inequality between countries. Essentially, he suggests, it would not then matter where a person lived. By contrast, reflect on the *present* level of inequality between rich and poor societies: in this case a person's home country 'determines everything'. The data for Denmark and Ethiopia, he adds, do not overlap at all. A person born in Denmark almost certainly has an income above the global average, while someone born in Ethiopia almost certainly has an income lower than that average. Milanovic (2015) found that the country where a person lives explains two-thirds of the variation in income differences between all the people on the planet. Where a person lives is the most important factor in their income. Until recently, very few people migrated to other countries, 97 per cent living in the countries in which they were born.

The chains linking absolute and/or relative poverty to premature death or sickness are complex; nor is it easy to generalise across national or community boundaries since economic infrastructures and political and cultural superstructures vary enormously. The concept of asset flows introduced earlier can still serve a useful function here, but its application is undeniably structurally and culturally dependent. But Hyde and Rosie (2012) offer an interesting starting point for our analysis. They rethink epidemiological transition theory (ETT) in light of

Wallerstein's world systems theory. ETT, they contend, suffers from a 'state-centric, methodologically nationalist approach'. Originally formulated in 1971, Abdel Omran's ETT has attracted considerable attention and triggered many studies and discussions. 'Conceptually,' he wrote, 'the theory of epidemiological transition focuses on the complex change in patterns of health and disease *and* on the interactions between these patterns and their demographic, economic and sociologic determinants and consequences' (Omran, 1971: 510). ETT starts from the fundamental premiss that mortality is a crucial factor in population dynamics. He then discerns a long-term shift in mortality and disease patterns of the kind charted in Chapter One, namely, the replacement of pandemics of infection by degenerative and 'man-made' disease and causes of death. This shift most profoundly affected children and, reflecting gender relations, young women. 'The shifts in health and disease patterns that characterize the epidemiologic transition are closely associated with the demographic and socioeconomic transition that constitute the modernization complex' (Omran, 1971: 532). Variations in the pattern, pace and the determinants and sequelae of population change suggest three models of the epidemiologic transition: the 'classic or Western model', the 'accelerated model' and the 'contemporary or delayed model'. Thus, the ETT is rooted in successive shifts from 'the age of pestilence and famine' through 'the age of receding pandemics' to 'the age of degenerative and man-made disease'. What is required of non-Western societies *stuck in neophyte stages of the modernisation process* is further (capitalist) development. It is an argument concerning which scepticism was expressed earlier in this volume. Hyde and Rosie rightly note that ETT assumes that what happened in the West will inevitably happen elsewhere; *and* that each nation is an independent actor free from interference.

The pioneer of world systems theory, Immanual Wallerstein, did not sign up to modernisation or development theory. His contention was that there have so far existed two types of world system: 'world-empires', such as the Roman and Han China Empires, were expansive bureaucratic structures with a single political centre and an axial division of labour, but multiple cultures; the 'world-economy', by contrast, is characterised by a large axial division of labour with multiple political centres and multiple cultures. The transition to a (Eurocentric) capitalist world-economy marked a turning point for Wallerstein. According to his framework it led to a subsequent world split into three zones: the core, the semi-periphery and the periphery. As Hyde and Rosie (2012: 117) summarise: 'Countries in the core were the developed, industrialised economies and those in the periphery are the "underdeveloped" economies, typically reliant on the export of raw materials to the core. Thus the world system operates as a set of mechanisms that redistributes resources from the periphery to the core.'

Countries in the core are economically and politically dominant and those in the periphery are economically and politically dominated. The semi-periphery comprises those countries edging towards industrialisation and diversification but which remain non-dominant in global trade, typically exporting more to the peripheral states and importing more from the core states.

Core countries might be expected to exhibit a number of common features: to be the most economically diversified, wealthy and powerful countries; to have strong central governments with a strong state and a sufficient tax base to allow for an infrastructure conducive to a strong economy; to be highly industrialised and to produce manufactured goods rather than raw materials for export; to specialise increasingly in the information, finance and service industries; to be innovators in new technologies and industries; to have a strong bourgeoisie and an organised working class; and to have significant means of influence over nations in the (semi) periphery while themselves remaining relatively independent of external control. In contrast, countries in the periphery typically have weak industrial bases and tend to be dependent on a small number of commodities, mainly primary goods and/or raw materials. They often have weak governments with disarticulated state structures. They have characteristically large informal and agricultural workforces, low rates of formal schooling and literacy and high levels of inequality, with wealth largely concentrated among small elites (Hyde and Rosie, 2012: 117).

The question Hyde and Rosie pose for themselves concerns the degree to which a sum of ETT and world systems theory might yield more than either of its parts. Exercising an appropriate degree of caution, the authors look at all-cause mortality in relation to trade dependency, and then build on this analysis to consider the proportion of deaths due to communicable, maternal, perinatal and nutritional diseases. They focus on West Africa as a region of anticipated high population growth and therefore a likely significant reflector of disease tendencies. Drawing on a substantial if diverse empirical literature they discern several distinctive periods. The first extensive period runs from BCE and encompasses the major African empires; the second marks the period of European discovery and the beginnings of European control (1500–1700); the third is characterised by the iniquities of the slave trade (1700–1800s); the fourth is that of European colonisation and decolonisation (1860–1960s); and the final and most recent period dates from the 1960s onwards. The gist of the authors' argument is that:

> there will be differences in both the size of the segments (bulk goods trade, prestige goods trade, political and military networks and the resulting information networks). The factors that influence such changes include of course the forms of trade, political and social relations in place that will change as the region is first incorporated as an external zone and peripheralised. (Hyde and Rosie, 2012: 124)

While world system theory delves into precisely these matters, it omits any account of the changing pattern of disease. ETT, on the other hand, pays only lip-service to the causal ramifications of economic and societal change for causes of death and the nature and distribution of disease.

Unsurprisingly, the historical West African data are not decisive; but they 'allow for' the authors' hypotheses that during the first period, from BCE until the end of the African kingdoms in the 15th century, trade in bulk and prestige goods was approximately in balance. This was due to the establishment and retention of regular trade patterns, though trade was not entirely 'self-contained' as that in salt, slaves and other goods occurred across the Sahara (and brought people into contact with other disease pools). In the second period of European exploration, the lines of information of the system changed, which led to changes in goods traded within the world system of the time. As European supercargoes became established, developing trade in palm oil from the 16th century, so trade in bulk goods declined and trade in prestige goods increased. This in turn led to an expansion in the movement of people. The consolidation of the slave trade and the peripheralisation of West Africa in the European world system amplified this process and was associated with a rise of sleeping sickness. Subsequently, in the colonial period, there began a significant movement of people from the northern part of the region to the cities of the south such as Lagos, which is one of the fastest growing cities in Africa. Part trade-related, this urban migration prompted a rise in diseases associated with poor sanitation and lack of clean water supplies.

As a representation and illustration of their thesis, Hyde and Rosie cite Steverding (2008: 5) on the Congo:

> Other factors that affected the epidemiology of sleeping sickness in the first half of the last century are the socio-economic conditions created during the colonisation of Africa. An excellent example of this is the sleeping sickness epidemic in the north-central Uele district of the former Belgian Congo, now known as the Democratic Republic of Congo. Colonisation of this region in the first decade of the 19th century was protracted and brutal. Large numbers of people were displaced and many of them experienced famine. This created an ideal environment for spreading the disease and sleeping sickness became increasingly entrenched and epidemic in this region over the next 15 years. It was not until the mid-1920s that medical services were introduced in the Uele district by the colonial powers.

As this quotation references, the African continent has long been – and continues to be – plagued by intermittent but persistent warfare. The increase of political-military conflict after decolonisation has led to 13 million deaths through warfare and starvation. Hyde and Rosie also comment on the development of the oil-refining industry. Considering this in light of their advocacy of a world system perspective, they focus specifically on Nigeria, which they argue has reverted from a mixed export provider of bulk goods to reliance on a single export – oil. Much of the profit has been drained off and the Delta region, they note, is poorer than the rest of the country. The observable increase in cancers and diarrhoeal illnesses that comprise major causes of death in the area was possibly exacerbated by the activities of the private militias hired by the oil companies. The authors' key point remains, however, namely that a significant shift in a pattern of trade in one commodity has emerged alongside a shift in disease types. And in this context they conclude by commending tracking the impacts of major transnational companies on the West African region, extending, for example, to the study of clean-up operations from toxic wastes and the impacts on health of export zones used to handle toxic materials.

A global perspective

Hyde and Rosie make an interesting and compelling case for combining macro-sociology and epidemiology via their investigation of ETT, both underwritten by and informed by world system theory. They challenge Omran's state-centrism by insisting on the salience of 'the global arena' and processes of globalisation. It has not been possible here, and will not be in the following chapter on climate change, to explore in detail the economic and social structures and cultures of multiple semi- and peripheral countries, but hopefully enough has been said already to make the case for the inter- as well as intranational investigation of population health and health inequality. But there is more that must be said here.

It is not just that population health and health inequalities require a global perspective. This is true also of health care systems and health interventions. The advent of COVID, following in the footsteps of pandemics throughout the ages, has shown why, and the extent to which, this is the case. Ahmed et al (2021) conducted a cross-sectional electronic survey of 928 health (57 per cent) and non-health professionals in six languages from 66 countries, with respondents recruited via email, social media and website posting. Respondents were then asked to score 'inhibitors' or 'facilitators' impacting country response to COVID from seven domains: political, economic, sociological, technological, ecological, legislative and wider industry. Descriptive and thematic analysis was then used to appraise free text responses. The study resulted in the development of a 103-item tool for guiding rapid situational assessment for pandemic planning.

As far as the political domain was concerned, lack of strategy and of detailed plans were typically seen as 'allowing politics to take primacy in decision-making and politicisation of the pandemic'. This is entirely consonant with the account of the UK response offered in Chapter Five, where emergency executive governmental powers were assumed, resulting in a surge in state authoritarianism. The principal criticisms were not of specific political parties but rather of individual leaders and leadership. Particular mention was made of the importance of transparency and trust. The timing of the pandemic in relation to the election cycle was also perceived as important: when elections were imminent, decisions were seen as driven by the need for short-term popularity.

Across high-, middle- and low-income countries disparities and inequities permeated almost every aspect of respondents' comments. Socio-economic conditions that older people lived in were recorded as barriers to effective responses, especially where informal support networks were weak and there were gaps in social services. Economic vulnerability impaired the public's ability to adopt protective measures, either voluntarily or in compliance with national policies. This, the authors report, links with 'inclusivity of vulnerable groups in mitigation plans' under the political domain. The challenges facing health care workers struggling to sustain themselves and their families in the face of economic precarity was an inhibitor, just as it was for the general population and for patients.

In what the authors designated the sociological domain, negative effects included declines in mental health wellbeing, largely from physical and social isolation, most notably among vulnerable groups. More positively, opportunities arose for changes in social norms and behaviours. The significance of the technological domain was appraised largely in terms of the ability to implement and scale up technology. However, while technology was noted as a facilitator for communication and e-health, this was counterbalanced by the potential for the spread of misinformation. Some respondents noted the tension between evidence-based policy and political or policy-based evidence. In the ecological domain, raised awareness of the risks attendant on pandemics in general and COVID in particular was mentioned in positive terms, as was a dip in air pollution levels. Negative impacts included risks to food security and agriculture and the increased use of disposable products. In the domain of legislation there was an emphasis on legislative inconsistency attributed to fragmentation between central and local governments, while a failure to implement legislation, sometimes exacerbated by a lack of available structures to enforce it, proved a barrier across several domains. Social norms were salient here too.

Corruption was cited as a barrier, including political and economic forms of corruption. Indeed, responses to the pandemic were impeded in the presence of endemic corruption. The pandemic was seen as creating opportunities for corruption and political opportunism. As one respondent put it: 'The government took advantage of the moment to monopolise everything in the executive branch and inactivate the Judiciary and Parliament. ... We have an undemocratic, authoritarian and corrupt government.' One of the lessons of this study, epitomised in this comment on corruption, is that it gives the lie to the politically expedient presumption in many high-income Western countries that the barriers to rational and effective policy-making with regard to pandemics in low-income, putatively under- or undeveloped countries are not exclusive to those countries and cannot be dismissed either as a function of local internal failure or as amenable to local internal correction. Witness here the deficits apparent in the UK government's COVID response, including political corruption, opportunism and incompetence, discussed in Chapter Five.

If the overriding theme of this chapter is that no country exists or can be studied in isolation, an offshoot is that measures taken to address population health and inequalities in health and health care in one country – notably in Wallerstein's core – can have significant ramifications for countries lying in his semi- or peripheral zones. Thus, in the unlikely event of the kinds of policies commended by the World Health Organization and Marmot in the UK being implemented there, in rentier capitalism this would almost certainly involve the extraction of an unacceptable price in other parts of the globe. The continuing orthodox neoliberal emphasis on national economic growth, currently promoted as the answer to the UK's cost of living crisis, brings with it the prospect of ramping up political domination and economic exploitation elsewhere. But in no sphere is the requirement to 'think global' more apparent than that of climate change associated with the Anthropocene.

SEVEN

Planet Earth

It is largely a function of sociology's divisions into specialisms that studies of population health and health inequalities tend, with a small but growing number of honourable exceptions, to be conducted in terms of individual nation states; and that phenomena like climate change tend also to be explored in an academic silo. In this chapter it is argued that the era of the Anthropocene has compelled a global orientation too long neglected or denied in the fields of health and health care. At the start of the last chapter, different if provisional views on the beginning of the Anthropocene were noted. While as yet there is no consensus, a team of scientists has recently affirmed the existence of a new geological time period marking the start of humanity's impact on the planet. While humans began to have an impact on the planet a while ago, with the rise of widespread farming and later the Industrial Revolution, these developments remained geographically restricted. Colin Waters, representing the Anthropocene Working Group (AWG), has maintained that the Anthropocene is 'visible globally' in the top sediment layer of the Earth's surface, starting in the 1950s. The AWG declares that the Anthropocene is marked by the appearance of plutonium and other indicators of the surge in human activity typically called 'the great acceleration'. Other 'markers' include the increasing consumption of fossil fuels, the greater use of nitrogen fertilisers and enhanced global trade spreading species across the planet and homogenising the plant and animal life of the planet. The AWG is focusing on Crawford Lake in Canada as a monitoring site. While some scientists still insist we are yet to leave the

Holocene period, others deploy a different nomenclature for the emergence of the Anthropocene, including the Capitalocene and even the Proletariocene.

Setting these disputes to one side, we can now agree on the nature and extent of recent climate change and its genesis in human activities. Ten of the warmest years since records were first kept 143 years ago have occurred since 2010. Although warming is not taking place uniformly across the plant, the upward trend in the globally averaged temperature shows that more areas are warming than cooling. The combined land and ocean temperature has increased at an average of 0.14 degree Fahrenheit (0.08 degree Celsius) per decade since 1880. However, the increase since 1981 has been more than twice as fast: 0.32 degree Fahrenheit (0.18 degree Celsius). At the time of writing, July 2023, we are on the verge of the hottest temperature ever recorded on Earth. The extent of future warming will be dependent on how much carbon dioxide (CO_2) and other greenhouse gases we emit in coming decades. Fossil fuels – coal, oil and gas – are by far the largest contributors to global climate change, accounting for over 75 per cent of global greenhouse gas emissions and nearly 90 per cent of all CO_2 emissions. As greenhouse gas emissions blanket the Earth, they trap the Sun's heat. This leads to global warming and climate change. Presently, using 2022 data, our activities – burning fossil fuels and clearing forests – add about 11 billion metric tonnes of carbon (equivalent to a little over 40 billion tonnes of CO_2) to the atmosphere each year. As this is more carbon than natural processes can remove, atmospheric CO_2 increases each year. Current models predict that if yearly emissions continue to increase as rapidly as they have since 2000, by the end of the 21st century global temperature will be at least 5 degrees Fahrenheit warmer than the 1901–60 average (and possibly as much as 10.2 degrees warmer) (NOAA, 2023).

As noted, Beck (1982, 1999) was prescient among sociologists in announcing the advent of 'risk society', arguing that the nature and threat attending contemporary risks have taken on a new and more threatening dimension. Moreover, they show a 'boomerang effect'. There is no escape: they come back to haunt those responsible for their generation. While there is truth in this observation, as with climate change, what was perhaps underplayed by Beck was the enduring tendency for these novel risks to most imperil the poorest people inhabiting low-income or peripheral countries. However, as Box 7.1 illustrates, the principal 'natural' consequences of climate change represent a significant risk also to citizens of the UK and other European countries.

Box 7.1: The natural consequences of climate change in Europe

High temperatures: this will lead to more frequent extremes, such as heatwaves, associated with increased mortality. The most vulnerable, such as the elderly and infants, will be most severely affected. High temperatures may also cause a shift in the distribution of climate zones, in the process redistributing plant and animal species. Enhanced numbers of pests and invasive species and, in consequence, a higher number of certain human diseases are likely. The yields and viability of agriculture and livestock, or the capacity of ecosystems to provide important services, such as the supply of clean water and cool and clean air, could be diminished.

Drought and wildfires: several European countries are already confronted by more frequent, severe and lengthy droughts. Droughts, products of a combination of lack of precipitation and more evaporation, differ from temporary deficits in water scarcity. Water scarcity refers to the structural year-round lack of fresh water due to the over-consumption of water. Droughts have knock-on effects, for example on transport infrastructure, agriculture, forestry, water supply and biodiversity. They reduce water levels in rivers and ground water, stunt tree and crop growth, increase pest attacks and fuel wildfires. It is predicted that with a global average temperature increase of 3 degrees Celsius droughts in Europe will occur twice as often. This would enhance the risk of wildfires, especially in the Mediterranean region.

Availability of fresh water: as the planet heats up, rainfall patterns change, evaporation increases, glaciers melt and sea levels rise, all of which affect the availability of fresh water. Water quality is expected to diminish with the spread of toxic algae and bacteria. Forty per cent of Europe's water comes from the Alps, so changes in snow and glacier dynamics and patterns of rainfall may lead to temporary water shortages across Europe. Changes to river flows due to drought may also affect inland shipping and the production of hydroelectric power.

Floods: climate change is expected to increase precipitation, which may lead to fluvial (river) flooding; and extreme rainfall is likely to lead to pluvial flooding (that is, without any body of water overflowing). River flooding is already a common occurrence in Europe. Heavy rainstorms are projected to become more common and more intense due to high temperatures, leading to more flash floods.

Sea level rise and coastal areas: the sea level has risen over the course of the 20th century and has accelerated over the last few decades. This is mostly due to thermal expansion of the oceans because of warming, but melting ice from glaciers and the Antarctic ice sheet is also contributing. Around 30 per cent of the EU population lives within 50 kilometres of the coast, and in areas that generate over 30 per cent of the EU's total GDP. There are growing risks of coastal flooding and erosion, and of seawater pushing into and contaminating underground water tables.

Biodiversity: the speed of climate change is already affecting plant and animal species via their behaviour and lifecycles (phenology), and in their abundance and distribution, community composition, habitat structure and ecosystem processes. Changes of land use and other resources are resulting in habitat fragmentation and loss, over-exploitation, pollution of air and water and soil, and the spread of invasive species.

Soils: climate change is likely to reduce organic matter and aggravate erosion, salination, soil diversity loss, landslides, desertification and flooding. Extreme precipitation events, fast melting snow or ice, high river discharges and increased droughts will all influence soil degradation. Deforestation and activities such as agriculture and skiing will also have an effect. Saline soils are expected to increase in coastal areas as a result of saltwater intrusion from the seaside because of rising sea levels and intermittent low river discharges.

Inland water: significant changes in water availability across Europe are predicted, especially in southern and south-eastern Europe, leading to water scarcity. Water temperature is a vital parameter for determining the overall health of aquatic ecosystems because aquatic organisms have a specific range of temperatures they can tolerate. The water temperatures of rivers and lakes are increasing and ice cover decreasing, in the process affecting water quality and freshwater ecosystems.

Marine environment: the physical and biological makeup of the oceans is shifting with climate change, affecting the geographical distribution of fish. Increasing sea temperature might also enable alien species to expand into regions where they could not previously survive. Ocean acidification, for example, will have an impact on a number of calcium carbonate-secreting organisms. These changes will have unavoidable impacts on coastal and marine ecosystems, with major social-economic consequences for many regions.

What the contents of Box 7.1 graphically illustrate is that climate change is of compelling importance across the globe and threatens even core or high-income countries as well as low-income or peripheral countries. The reach of its multiple tentacles, and therefore the degree of its threat, is of deep and immediate concern.

Anthropocene, Capitalocene or Proletariocene?

Despite both the coalescence of scientific views on climate change and the insistent intergovernmental rhetoric on the urgent need for action, it remains apparent that curtailing the use of fossil fuels has proven, and continues to prove, too difficult a challenge. The Paris Agreement at COP21 on 12 December 2015 was signed by 196 parties and entered into force on 4 November 2016. Its overarching goals were to hold the increase in global average temperature to well below 2 degrees Celsius above pre-industrial levels and to pursue efforts to limit the temperature increase to 1.5 per cent above pre-industrial levels. In the period after this, the importance of limiting global warming to 1.5 degrees Celsius by the end of this century has been emphasised. Crossing the 1.5 degrees Celsius threshold, the UN's Intergovernmental Panel on Climate Change has insisted, brings severe risks of the kind foretold in Box 7.1. Indeed, rising temperatures are already killing thousands of people. One study showed that up to 61,000 people died in 2022 as a direct result of heat waves across Europe (see Blakeley, 2023). In the USA, extreme heat is already the 'top annual weather-related killer'. Air pollution, too, is killing people, causing 6.7 million premature deaths each year. Extreme weather events such as floods, wildfires and droughts are more common – having increased fivefold over the last 50 years – and have led to two million deaths and $4.3 trillion worth of economic damage. Only too predictably, more than 90 per cent of these deaths have occurred in the semi- and peripheral countries located in the Global South: 'those forced to bear the consequences of global warming largely caused by the global North and those least able to bear the economic and health consequences' (see Blakeley, 2023).

To limit global warming to 1.5 degrees Celsius, greenhouse gas emissions must peak before 2025 at the latest and decline by 2030. COP28 is due to be convened in Dubai in November/ December of 2023 and will focus on a stocktake of progress made since COP21. Its president is Al Jaber, who will call for an urgent and immediate phasing down of fossil fuels even as he retains his role as chief of the United Arab Emirates national oil company, Adnoc (Harvey, 2023). The omens are not good. Nor is the UK government responding with any sense of an imminent crisis. 'It's hard', Bill McGuire (2023) writes, 'not to wonder if the government is not living on another planet'. He continues: 'With global emissions needing to fall by half within seven years, it is now practically impossible for us to stay this side of the 1.5 degrees Centigrade dangerous climate change guardrail.'

Referring to the UK government's recent statement of intent, he observes that while it is big on consultation, research, monitoring, building frameworks and gathering information, 'there is a failure to recognise that these are luxuries whose time has come and gone'. There is further evidence of governmental laggardness in the fact that fossil fuels have received £20 billion more support in the UK than renewables since 2015. Moreover, one-fifth of the money given directly to the fossil fuel industry was to support new extraction and mining (Horton, 2023). Furthermore, at the time of writing (July 2023) UK Prime Minister Sunak has not just cut back on green targets but announced that the government has approved licences for over 100 new oil drilling initiatives off the coast of Scotland, arguing, to the disbelief and dismay of climate activists, that this is perfectly consistent with the UK's net zero commitments. Murphy (2023) castigates Sunak's decision, suggesting that there are three principal reasons for it, each representing a form of appeasement. The first reason, he argues, is to appease his Conservative backbenchers. The second is to appease the right-wing media, 'who are totally out of sync with the population of the UK on this issue'. And the third is to appease the oil companies:

It remains the case today that they, along with a range of other big businesses, and particularly global finance whose fortunes are intimately related to oil because of the funding that they supply to it, remain dedicated to extracting oil and gas from the planet, whatever the consequences for humankind.

It has also emerged that Sunak's Conservative Party has received millions of pounds in donations from 'climate deniers' and others with interests in the fossil fuel industry (Garton-Crosby, 2023). Furthermore, it has been claimed that Sunak and his family are themselves intimately linked to the fossil fuel industry through his wife Akshata Murty's stake in the transnational IT services firm Infosys, one of whose top clients is oil giant Shell. This information was made public after a High Court ruling obtained by the Good Law Project. Akshata Murty may be a minority shareholder in Infosys, owning a £690 million stake in the firm owned by her father, but she collected an estimated £11.5 million in dividend payments from Infosys over the past year (see Ahmed, 2022). It goes without saying that this is consonant with the class/command dynamic.

This is occurring at a time when southern Mediterranean countries are experiencing raised temperatures of 40 degrees Celsius plus and a spate of wildfires causing mass evacuations and infrastructural and economic devastation, especially among the Greek Islands. It is in this context that a report by leading climate scientists should be interpreted. The first week in July 2023 saw the temperature records shattered around the world, not just in the southern Mediterranean but also in the western USA and Mexico and China. These scientists calculate that greenhouse gas emissions made the heatwaves 2.5 degrees Celsius hotter in Europe, 2 degrees Celsius hotter in North America and 1 degree Celsius hotter in China than if human activity had not changed the global atmosphere. UN Secretary General António Guterres is on record as warning that:

> 'Humanity is in the hot seat. For vast parts of North America, Asia, Africa and Europe, it (2023) is a cruel summer. For the entire planet, it is a disaster. And for

scientists, it is unequivocal – humans are to blame. All this is entirely consistent with predictions and repeated warnings. The only surprise is the speed of the change. Climate change is here, it is terrifying, and it is just the beginning. The era of global warming has ended; the era of global boiling has arrived.' (Niranjan, 2023)

The authors of the UN-based report from the Intergovernmental Panel on Climate Change deliver a no less stark warning: 'There is a rapidly closing window of opportunity to secure a liveable and sustainable future for all.' They add: 'The choices and actions implemented in this decade [that is, by 2030] will have impacts now and for thousands of years.' Lives and livelihoods are already being lost, especially in the semi- and peripheral countries of the world system. The report reiterates that greenhouse gas emissions *must* peak 'at the latest' before 2025, followed by 'deep global reductions'. However, global emissions rose again to set a new record in 2022 (see Carrington, 2023).

As far as the global economic context is concerned, despite a dip during COVID, the world experienced a rapid economic recovery driven by unprecedented fiscal and monetary stimulus and a relatively fast, if predictably uneven, roll out of vaccines. The recovery of energy demand by 2021 was compounded by adverse weather and energy market conditions, which led to more coal burning despite renewable power generation registering its largest annual growth. There was a 6 per cent increase in CO_2 emissions in 2021, which was in line with the jump in global economic output of 5.9 per cent (marking the strongest coupling of CO_2 emissions with GDP since 2010). Coal accounted for over 40 per cent of the overall growth in global CO_2 emissions in 2021 and now stands at an all-time high (for additional data, see the report of the International Energy Agency (2022)). As far as the UK is concerned, the increase in emissions in 2021, post-COVID, were primarily due to the increase in transport post-lockdowns (responsible for 26 per cent of all UK greenhouse gas emissions in 2021).

In his *Climate Change as Class War*, Matthew Huber (2022) does not pull his punches. Picking up on the concept of a 'just transition' he insists that the focus needs to be on 'worker power' and bemoans the fact that so much discussion of climate change and greenhouse gas emissions, extending to 'environmental politics' – even on 'the left' – omits any real analysis of the relevance of the class struggle over industrial production: 'For much of the left, climate and environment struggle is a "movement" distinct from class-based movements. Tensions between these movements is often constructed as a zero-sum game between "jobs" and "environment". Indeed, trade union leaders have often echoed these divisions' (Huber, 2022: 69). The climate issue, he argues, is a class issue in three fundamental ways. First, the – presently failing – climate struggle needs to focus on *production*. If we are to effectively address climate change and ecological breakdown, even in contemporary 'post-industrial' societies, we must acknowledge that the entire human relationship to the natural world is, at its core, a relationship of production, encompassing how we produce food, energy, housing and the other basics of life. A production-centred approach 'means we need to focus our organising energy against the particular class fraction that controls the production of energy from fossil fuels and other industrial carbon-intensive industries like steel, cement … and nitrogen fertiliser' (Huber, 2022: 4).

Key here, deploying my terminology, are the capital monopolists who buy power from national politicians to shape policy. The privatisation of water in the UK over three decades ago provides one of numerous examples of rentier capitalism writ large. Privatisation, it was promised, would usher in a new era of investment, more competitive bills and improved water quality. Enter Macquarie. Macquarie was set up as a subsidiary of the British bank Hill Samuel and Co in 1969, prior to obtaining an Australian banking licence in the 1980s. Its robustness currently stands in stark contrast to the impoverished state of Thames Water, which suffered an increase in debt from £3.4 billion to £10.8 billion during the Macquarie consortium-led ownership from 2006 to 2017. Estimates have put the dividends paid to underlying investors, including itself, for Thames Water at £2.7 billion over the 11-year period it oversaw 'the asset'. The Macquarie group has been tagged the 'millionaire factory'. Nick O'Kane, head of Macquarie's commodities and global markets division 'earned' Australian $57.6 million during the last financial year (up from Australian $32.8 million the previous year) (Barrett, 2023). Meanwhile Thames Water, which had no debt prior to privatisation, is presently the most indebted water company with leverage exceeding 80 per cent, most of which was acquired during Macquarie's tenure. Ironically, Macquarie sold its financial stake in Thames Water in 2017, the same year it took over the government's Green Investment Bank for £2.3 billion. It was a well-timed opt-out. Days after its exit Thames Water was hit by what was, at the time, a record fine of £20.3 million linked to huge leaks of untreated sewage in 2013 and 2014. Extraordinarily, Macquarie was subsequently permitted back into the UK water industry, buying a majority share in Southern Water.

It should be apparent that what is of foremost importance is not so much the individuals who qualify as capital monopolists, but rather *the structures that define, sustain and protect these substitutable 'greedy bastards'*. As Marx's analysis of 'capital personified' makes clear, the accumulation drive for surplus value by individual capitalists is not a choice, but a structural necessity impelled by what he called external 'coercive laws of competition' (Huber, 2022: 106).

Second, we must recognise that a specific class, the *professional class*, now dominates the climate movement. This class specialises in mental or cognitive labour and comprises a segment of the knowledge economy. This has two consequences. Professional-class climate politics 'fixates' on its own comfortable assumption that it is ideas that matter and thus sidesteps industrial production. And relatedly, it centres its politics on knowledge rather than material struggle. While it promotes consideration of system change, climate justice and de-growth, it offers little by way of a strategy for building an effective mass movement to defeat the fossil fuel industry. In the UK, active campaign groups such as 'Stop Oil' might fall into this category. Climate politics in the USA (and the UK), Huber argues, primarily appeals to a minority of the population, roughly 'the upper third of the educated and credentialised classes'. It is not irrelevant to note that this minority has, in large measure, been able to ride out the growing material and social inequalities of rentier capitalism and remains sheltered from the worst effects of the 2023 cost of living crisis in the UK.

Huber's (2022: 6–7) third point here is that we do indeed need a mass movement to secure change. And only the working class, broadly defined, has the capacity to achieve this kind of mass movement. He includes within his definition of the working class the ecological separation from the 'conditions of life', which compels workers to survive via the market and without the resources available to the professional class. He sees working-class power as rooted in three factors. The first is the fact that it encompasses the vast majority of the population, 'meaning any *democratic or majoritarian* approach to climate action must build a working-class coalition'. Second, 'its strategic location at the point of production gives it structural power over the source of capital's profits and social reproduction generally'. It follows that working-class power is most effective during periods of strikes and disruption that put capitalists on the back foot. Third, as economic precarity or insecurity defines working-class life, its members have a fundamental material interest in transforming the relations of production. But he prudently adds: '[T]he defeats of Green New Deal candidates like Jeremy Corbyn and Bernie Sanders remind us that such "interests" are not pre-given, but must be organised through durable working-class institutions like political parties, unions, and media infrastructure.'

While much of the debate over climate politics and energy policy has been focused on the fossil fuel industry, a number of scientists and commentators have pointed out that the electric power sector is the 'lynchpin' of any decarbonisation strategy. While any union engagement on climate will tend to focus on the lot and futures of workers in the fossil fuel economy, Huber argues that the 'electric sector' represents a 'neutral technological system' that already generates electricity from many – often clean – sources, not just via fossil fuels. An effective form of climate politics should not just stress the negative programme of destroying the fossil fuel industry, but also a positive politics of cleaning up electricity. The current predilection for an 'electrifying everything strategy' should: (i) clean up the existing electric power sector, and (ii) significantly expand clean electricity production to absorb the new demand from the transport, heating and industrial sectors.

Building on this, Huber then contends that a working-class climate strategy should pinpoint the electric power sector. His argument is USA-based. He notes that the electric utility sector in the USA, although largely run by private or 'investor-owned' utilities, is already subject to public oversight and political contestation. As Strauss and Mapes (2012) write: 'Many traditional labour union concerns – including ensuring adequate staffing levels and safe working conditions – are intimately intertwined with a utility's ability to provide an adequate service.' This has resonance with the UK electricity sector. Workers, Huber suggests, might readily link their more immediate safety concerns to a more far-reaching global vision of safe levels of emissions on a planetary scale. Furthermore, workers in the electric industry literally possess 'power' over the economy as a whole. Their sector is central both to capital accumulation and the social reproduction of everyday life ('when the power goes out, people notice'). In a statement that echoes people's circumstances during the cost of living crisis in the UK, Huber (2022: 236) writes:

> Speaking theoretically, a strike in the electricity sector would effectively shut down society, creating the effect of a general strike, given that economic activity is impossible without electricity. ... Since we have ceded electricity distribution mostly to private investor-owned utilities demanding high rates to support their 'fair' rates of return, there is already an existing reservoir of mass working-class anger toward utility companies.

A final point here is that the electric sector is already one of the most highly unionised sectors globally as well as in the US. In a nutshell, Huber advocates a 'rank-and-file strategy' starting out in and subsequently expanding from the electric sector. In this respect the 'proletarian class', rather than the higher profile and newsworthy professional class, is deemed the only realistic agent for transformatory change. These are matters for further and deeper consideration in the chapters that follow.

The contention at the conclusion of the previous chapter was that material and social inequality should no longer be studied and addressed as national phenomena but should adopt a global frame. Securing a reduction in the maldistribution of those asset flows conducive to good health and longevity in a country like the UK should not come at the price of enhanced neo-imperialistic economic and political exploitation and domination elsewhere. Introducing the quintessentially urgent challenge of climate change into the equation further complicates an already complicated arena of research, policy and practice: how to reconcile prioritising reducing global greenhouse gas emissions without compromising an already difficult and expanded inequalities agenda? Ian Gough (2017: 195) articulates this problematic as follows:

> [E]liminating poverty on a world scale can only be squared with planetary sustainability if the current model of economic growth is abandoned. If the business-as-usual were used to eliminate poverty it would devastate the planet. All strategies to eliminate global poverty are untenable unless the poor get a bigger slice of the whole cake, but there are limits to its expansion because of global constraints on emissions.

Gough advocates the introduction of 'need based criteria' in the form of a measure of what he calls the 'emissions efficiency of wellbeing'. But a further quandary requires to be confronted, namely, the salience of war for global, national and individual health.

EIGHT

War

The character of war has always shifted along with technological and societal change. After the Second World War and thus far in the 21st century, notwithstanding the current conflict in Ukraine and in and around the Gaza Strip, direct wars between major powers have been absent. Rather, these powers have either waged proxy wars or attacked smaller countries. The weapons at their disposal have grown exponentially in their destructiveness, which largely accounts for their reluctance to engage each other directly. In terms of numbers, by the time of the advent of post-1970s' rentier capitalism, annual deaths from warfare had reduced to 'the low hundreds of thousands' (fewer than those who die from traffic accidents) (Dyer, 2021). This is not to minimise the chronic conflict zones in south-western Asia, Africa, the Middle East and elsewhere, all of which have led, and continue to lead, to countless deaths of troops and citizens. But the inclusion of this chapter on war reflects its role in what is likely to be a rapidly growing family of threats to the very idea of a healthy society; and once again the omens are not good. Why is this?

Violent conflict has long characterised human society, for all that it is not plausible to refer to 'wars' in early hunter-gatherer bands, that is, prior to the emergence of more settled 'tribal' communities (see Box 1.1). Since then, the nature of war has evolved along with political and technological change. In the Occident, in the Fordist/welfare capitalism of the post-Second World War years and in rentier capitalism, war for combat forces and publics alike might be said to reflect what Norbert Elias' (1969), in a strict sociological sense, calls a 'civilising process'. In other words, the deployment of anonymous technologies such as missiles and drones has replaced much, if not all, brutal hand-to-hand bloodletting. Indeed, waiting in the wings are novel Lethal Autonomous Weapons Systems (LAWS), namely, robots 'free to make their own decisions'; these could be operational within the next decade. Modern warfare is sometimes referred to as 'fourth-generation warfare'. This denotes a form of war in which conflicts are complex, multifaceted, long-term and decentralised, with the boundaries between military and civil strategies significantly blurred (for example, media-led warfare). But all this is not for a moment to suggest that geopolitically dominant countries in the Global North, most notably the USA and in Europe, have been reticent in fighting, precipitating, sponsoring and exporting war across all its gory and pre-civilised formats. Major wars launched by the USA after the Second World War are those in Korea, Vietnam, Kosovo, Afghanistan and Iraq, while minor but active engagements occurred also in the Bay of Pigs, Grenada, Panama, the Persian Gulf, Bosnia and Herzegovina, north-west Pakistan, Somalia and Northeastern Kenya, Libya, Syria and the Yemeni Civil War. These conflicts witnessed the export too of massive – civilian as well as combatant – death and suffering.

If the USA has been the most active and belligerent major power in recent times, the role of the UK warrants special attention. The British military has used or threatened the use of military force more often in the postwar world than is commonly appreciated or understood. Declassified UK (2023) has documented 83 interventions by the UK armed forces since 1945, in 47 different countries. These engagements range from brutal colonial wars and covert operations to efforts to prop up favoured governments or to deter civil unrest. The use of force for overt invasions or armed attempts to overthrow governments include British Guiana (now Guyana) in 1953, Egypt in the 1950s, Iraq in 2003 and Libya in 2011. Of primary salience for the UK's postwar military history is its longstanding role as a colonial and hegemonic power and the deep and obstinate shadow it continues to cast on the contemporary world system; and it is this that affords a compelling point of departure for our brief excursus on the health-sapping structural, cultural and agential sequelae of war.

As one American commentator reminds us, 'at the height of the British Empire, just after the First World War, an island smaller than Kansas controlled roughly a quarter of the world's population and landmass' (Khilnani, 2022). To its architects and enforcers, each conquest was a moral victory; and imperial tutelage, 'often imparted through the barrel of an Enfield', delivered peoples from their pre-civilised or barbarian imprisonment. In *Legacy of Violence*, Caroline Elkins (2022) debunks this self-serving mythology. Her book sits on the shoulders of her previous path-breaking book disseminating her research on the brutal suppression of the Mau Mau movement in Kenya in the 1950s. She estimated a tally of up to 300,000 Mau Mau dead or missing. Following a High Court case, her research resulted in reparations to the 5,228 surviving Kenyans who, the British government was forced to accept, had been subject to years of systematic torture and abuse. Elkins argues that Britain was every bit as brutal as other colonial powers, even if it was better at concealing this fact.

As the only imperial power that remained a liberal democracy through the 20th century, Britain insisted it was distinct from other European colonial powers in its commitment to exporting the rule of law, Enlightenment principles and social progress to its colonies. As Elkins documents in meticulous detail, however, Britain utilised systematic violence on a scale comparable to its rivals. She shows how repression was visited on South Africa, India, Ireland and Palestine, and addresses it too in Malaya, Kenya, Cyprus and Aden. Brutality abroad went unchecked at home and was underpinned by the full force of law. She vividly recounts:

> The practice of blowing Indian sepoys from cannons after the 1857 uprising, the Maxim-gun slaughter of Mahdists in the eighteen-nineties, the use of concentration camps in the Boer wars, the massacre of peaceful protests in Amritsar, reprisal killings and the sacking of civilian property in Ireland: all this state-inflicted savagery was just the British Empire warming up. (See Khilnani, 2022)

For all its rhetoric about universal freedom and the like, British liberalism served the goals of empire by rationalising its domination and exploitation of other peoples. The British model of state violence, Elkin summarises, came wrapped in this 'velvet glove' of liberal reform. Well into the period following the Second World War, the heavy and bloody hand of British imperialism was felt across the globe.

Consider briefly the British strategy of detention, beatings, starvation, torture, forced hard labour, rape and castration designed to break the resistance of the Kikuyu, a Bantu-speaking people inhabiting the highland area of south-central Kenya who had been dispossessed by the British and subsequently enlisted during the Second World War to fight for them. Elkins explores this episode in detail in her *Imperial Reckoning*, published in 2005. She notes how in 1957 a British colonial governor, 'justifying' a brutal campaign, ironically named 'Operation Progress', told his superiors in London that 'violent shock' was the only way to break down hard core resisters. In excess of one million men, women and children were forced into barbed-wire bounded village compounds and concentration camps for 're-education'. The colony's attorney general at the time revealingly commented that this was 'distressingly reminiscent of conditions in Nazi Germany or Communist Russia'. Details like this are important because they both debunk and give the lie to obstinate myths of British benevolence overseas, and supply a vital historical background also to Britain's contemporary forms of what John Rex (1973) called 'internal colonialism'.

Britain's colonial past echoes through a contemporary British society that might still be represented in the guise of internal colonialism. It continues to have purchase in its own right as well as being filtered through the class/command, stigma/deviance, insider/outsider, elite/mass and party/populist dynamics listed earlier. Although members of ethnic minorities have contributed significantly to British society, too many of them only too often experience the discriminatory disadvantages attendant on poor class position and political disempowerment; are blamed for the structural and cultural circumstances in which they find themselves; are marginalised and 'othered' as outsiders; remain under-represented among elites; and are victimised in increasingly authoritarian and populist-oriented 'racism-for-votes' party politics. As Riley (2023) has shown in her *Imperial Island: A*

History of Empire in Modern Britain, the imperial mindset is alive and well, articulated in the jingoism of the Falklands War and regularly resuscitated since, for example in the tragedy of the Stephen Lawrence murder and its subsequent mishandling by a Metropolitan Police found to be 'institutionally racist', the Windrush deportations, Brexit and the current Conservative government's explicitly racist treatment of refugees and asylum seekers arriving across the English Channel in small, fragile boats. In these respects, Britain's historic warmongering overseas lives on in the present in the guise of internal colonialism or institutional racism. War, in other words, typically has deep and enduring consequences.

Thermonuclear war, the arms industry and corporate armies

Various other facets of war demand brief consideration at this point. 'Conventional' (non-nuclear) wars between nation states have been relatively rare since 1945, in large part due to the United Nations Charter's ban on changing borders. There have, however been a handful of significant failures, including the eight-year war between Iraq and Iran in the 1980s (prolonged by US and Russian aid to Saddam Hussein in the hope that he would destroy the revolutionary Islamic regime in Iran), plus 'great-power' moves such as the Soviet invasion of Afghanistan in 1979 and the US invasion of Iraq in 2003, both of which were illegal. At the time of writing, the ongoing Russian invasion of Ukraine must be appended to this list, as must the US and EU-armed Israeli war conducted against Palestinians in Gaza. Most of the conflict deaths over the last generation, however, have been the victims of civil wars – mainly in Africa – in which the UN has no mandate to interfere. Rural and urban guerrilla warfare have also been important and persistent themes, albeit with reduced effect in diminishing colonial and post-imperial contexts. But the era of the US/Soviet Cold War, ending with the dissolution of the Soviet Union, was primarily characterised, even defined by, the threat of a nuclear war; and for all that the Cold War has been concluded, Putin's invasion of Ukraine has reinvigorated concerns and debates about the nuclear threat. This threat is of vital concern to anyone committed to or interested in global health.

Strategies around nuclear arsenals have dominated great-power thinking for 75 years. Two 'quite small' bombs were dropped on Japanese cities in 1945 with devastating effect, and none have been deployed since. But the Cuban missile crisis in 1961 served to concentrate global and national government minds. Discussions about the likelihood and plausibility of a limited or contained nuclear conflict came to the fore and persist, including currently in relation to Ukraine. In the 1980s, at the height of the Cold War, a considerable body of research was conducted on the probable effects of an escalating nuclear confrontation, and the results were horrifying. As Carl Sagan commented in 1983: 'We have, by slow and imperceptible steps, been constructing a Doomsday Machine. Until recently, and then only by accident – no one even noticed. And we have distributed its triggers all over the Northern Hemisphere' (Sagan, 1983: 285).

One group of scientists utilised data from Mariner 9's observations of Mars and after a decade of multiple investigations published their findings in 1983. They concluded that a major nuclear exchange would cover the Northern Hemisphere, and possibly the entire planet,

> with a pall of smoke and dust that would plunge the surface into virtual darkness for up to six months. In the continental interiors, the surface temperature would drop by up to 40 degrees Centigrade (below the freezing point in any season) for a similar period. And when enough of the dust and soot particles drifted down from the stratosphere to let the sun's light back in, the destruction of the ozone layer by thermonuclear fireballs would let two or three times as much ultraviolet light reach the surface, causing blindness or lethal sunburn in exposed humans. (Dyer, 2021: 173)

This prospect of a 'nuclear winter' was worse even than the anticipated immediate loss of several hundred million lives, and yet more from famine and disease in the aftermath of a nuclear conflagration.

Arsenals, nuclear and conventional, must be manufactured and have unsurprisingly resulted in substantial trading. The UK's arms industry was the sixth largest exporter of major conventional weapons between 2012 and 2021 (behind the USA, Russia, France, China and Germany). Over the course of this decade, aircraft were the UK's principal arms export, making up 48 per cent of the total. The main arms deals are with the US, India, France, Germany, Italy, Israel, Oman, South Africa, Turkey, South Korea, the United Arab Emirates and Saudi Arabia; and arms manufactured in the UK include bombs, missiles, machine guns and fighter jets. But Britain's arms exports went on to double during 2022, to a record £8.5 billion, reflecting what were defined as 'growing geopolitical uncertainty' and the fallout from the ongoing Russian invasion of Ukraine. The UK's largest 'defence company' is BAE Systems, a transnational arms, security and aerospace company based in London with a revenue, in 2022, of £21,258 billion and an operating income of £2,384 billion. BAE was formed in 1999 with the purchase of and merger with Marconi Electronic Systems, the defence electronics and naval shipbuilding subsidiary of the General Electric Company, by British Aerospace, an aircraft, munitions and naval systems manufacturer. By 2017, BAE had become the biggest manufacturer in Britain. In short, there is a lot of money in arms *and in wars*. And as we have seen, money in the form of capital buys power to fashion policy. Labour Foreign Secretary Robin Cook, who resigned in protest over the illegal US/UK invasion of Iraq in 2003, said of his time in office under Tony Blair that he 'came to learn that the chairman of BAE appeared to have the key to the garden door to "Number 10". Certainly, I never knew No 10 to come up with any decision which would be incommoding to BAE' (Cook, 2017).

Corporate armies also play a pivotal role in the world system. There have for centuries existed mercenary fighters, but War on Want (2023), emphasising that war has long been a significant cause of poverty, has reported that Private Military and Security Companies (PMSCs) that sell security and military services at home and overseas have 'moved from the periphery of international politics into the corporate boardroom, becoming a normal part of the military sector'. The PMSC industry currently comprises hundreds of companies operating in more than 50 countries and offering their services to governments, international institutions and corporations. It is an industry that has expanded exponentially in recent years, not least in the aftermath of the illegal, UN-defying invasion of Iraq. Contracts in Iraq boosted the annual revenue of British PMSCs alone from £320 million in 2003 to more than £1.8 billion in 2004. War on Want quotes a report estimating that there are 48,000 mercenaries in Iraq. Income from the PMSC industry reached $100 billion in 2004. PMSCs play a significant role in enabling governments to cover their tracks and evade accountability. They are typically not accountable to governments or publics and in consequence permit governments to dissociate themselves and sidestep legal obstacles. War on Want assert that some major countries, such as the US and UK, 'would now struggle to wage war without PMSC partners'. Moreover, the lines between regular soldiers and PMSC employees has become blurred and the latter remain largely unregulated despite voiced concerns about the potential for human rights abuses.

War and health

It is obvious that war between or within nation states results in death and suffering. And it is no less apparent that a major nuclear conflict would threaten the very future viability of our and many other species. But it is important to document something of the known health impacts of armed conflict – in whatever of its many forms – on the health and wellbeing of those caught up in it. Every year many people are affected by explosive remnants of war (ERW); and this is true not only in areas of active conflict but in countries that have not been at war for decades. ERWs in Laos, for example, have injured or killed more than 50,000 people since the end of the Laotian Civil War in 1975. In 2015, landmines alone caused, on average, 18 casualties a day globally. The wide-ranging effects of ERWs on populations, with effects going on well beyond direct injuries to embrace impacts on livelihoods, mental health, public health and overall security, have been documented.

The contamination of private and public spaces experienced in Northern Syria, encompassing homes, fields, streets, schools and hospitals, impede the provision of functioning services and any return to more normal lives. ERWs also comprise a threat to public health via the destruction of water and sanitation infrastructures. Studies, Kate White and Sophie Désoulières (2023) pointedly argue in their review of the literature,

> should go beyond looking at the number of years of life lost to analysing the much broader effect on a society of living or having lived in an ERW-contaminated environment than that ascertained from just looking at the number of years of life lost. Findings from these studies should then provide an incentive to prioritise decontamination.

A number of other health sequelae of wars and conflicts require a mention. First, a word might be said of combatants themselves, many of whom cannot be said to have freely 'chosen' their engagement. Mortality rates in conventional warfare can be very high. The *daily* dead and wounded in a pre-20th century – or in Elias' strict sense of the term, 'pre-civilised' – battle often amounted to 40–50 per cent of the men engaged and was only rarely less than 20 per cent. The likely casualty toll in a single day has since plummeted, although the cumulative loss rate remains about the same. Dyer (2021: 31) argues, however, that the psychological impact of battle is now considerable:

> Troops are shelled every day, the enemy is always close, and they live amid constant death. This inexorably erodes men's faith in their own survival, and eventually destroys everybody's courage and will. 'Your courage flows at its outset with the fullest force and thereafter diminishes; perhaps if you are very brave it diminishes imperceptibly; but it does diminish … and it can never behave otherwise'.

The US Army calculated during the Second World War that almost every soldier, if he escaped death or wounds, would break down after 200–240 'combat days'. And then there is the matter of the long-term disabilities, psychological trauma and rehabilitation of the wounded and more fortunate survivors. At the time of writing, these words have a peculiar European resonance with regard to both Ukrainian and Russian forces involved in the current conflict.

The fighting in Ukraine, and more recently in Gaza, has also brought home the devastating consequences of warfare on civilian populations. This goes well beyond fatalities and injuries. There is an extensive research literature on this, but Goto and colleagues (2022) have provided an up-to-date summary of the health issues, with special reference to the experiences of children caught up in war zones, in the *Lancet*. War, they conclude, has both short- and long-term public health consequences. People can develop health problems stemming from the traumatic experience of war and scarcity of access to adequate health care. Moreover, war can affect people at any point of the life-course, and for extended periods of time. But given the overriding importance of the early years of a child's life, it is children, the authors contend, who are almost certainly most profoundly impacted by war. They cite research confirming that children exposed to war experience both higher mortality rates and an increased risk of becoming orphans; children faced with the toxic stresses of war could develop multiple mental health issues, including post-traumatic stress disorder, depression, anxiety, behavioural problems and suicidal behaviour, all of which are difficult to treat due to the scarcity or even absence of mental health resources in war zones; and children, and society, can be disadvantaged – the authors' word is 'crippled' – in subsequent years by hampering healthy development via severed early childhood education and exposure to toxic stress. Referring directly to the war in Ukraine, the authors state that this conflict constitutes a reminder of the wide-ranging and far-reaching damage that war can inflict. 'War', they state, 'is a public health emergency that spans numerous years.' They conclude with a demand on behalf of the International Society for Adolescent Psychiatry and Psychology, the International Association for Child and Adolescent Psychiatry and Allied Professions, the World Association for Infant Mental Health, and the Child and Adolescent Psychiatry Section of the

World Psychiatric Association that 'all fighting cease immediately and that all avenues for just and peaceful resolution of conflict be assertively pursued'.

It may seem unexpected, even incongruous, to include a chapter on warfare in a book on health. Indeed, the decision to do so was made late in the day. The rationale is that intra- and international inequality must be addressed within a broader global and macro-sociological context, and this involves the incorporation of accounts not only of longstanding issues of economic domination and exploitation but of climate change and conflict. This seems undeniable. Dyer (2021: 215) convincingly claims that a triad of changes are under way that could undo any modest political accomplishments: 'global heating, the rise of new great powers, and nuclear proliferation'. He expresses this concern in the following words:

> Rising global temperature will have disastrous effects on food production in the tropics and sub-tropics at least a generation before similar impacts are felt in the rich countries of the temperate latitudes. The consequence will be famines in those countries nearer to the equator and millions-strong waves of desperate refugees trying to get into the developed countries. The borders will slam shut, of course, but the only way to keep them shut against such numbers may be some form of 'exemplary' killing of those who try to breach them. The net result is likely to be a widespread breakdown in international cooperation (including cooperation in dealing with climate change), as it is difficult for countries to make arrangements and compromises when one country is killing another's citizens.

And all this while the world system is in the process of adjusting to the emergence of new great powers alongside the USA, namely China and India.

It is a difficult case to counter. Throughout this volume reference has intermittently been made to social and sociological theory, though it has been with a light touch. It is time now to justify and fortify the implicit assertion that theory matters. In the next chapter I revisit theories in the Marxist tradition. I offer a brief and simplified exposition of Marx's own perspective on capitalism, extending to his later and largely unpublished and unrecognised contributions on environmental threat, followed by an introduction to Jurgen Habermas' critical theory and Roy Bhaskar's critical realist approach to Marxism, and Margaret Archer's (non-Marxist) development of some of the latter's theories. In the chapter that follows on I focus on theories that directly confront the structural, cultural and agential obstacles that stand in the way of transformational societal change.

NINE

Why theory matters

We theorise like it or not. Any description of the natural or social worlds we inhabit, quite independently of its scientific status or level of subtlety, presumes an element of theory. None of us starts with a blank slate. We draw on a symbolic framework handed down and absorbed as if by osmosis from previous generations. We inherit a collection of language games or forms of life when we are socialised into a mix of lifeworld and expert perspectives. Society precedes us, for all that it neither exists independently of human activity nor is the product of it. *We are all where we start from.* But where we start from, whether as curious 'lay' citizens or as 'professional/expert' physicists, biologists or sociologists, is replete with theories that we have to take on board, with varying degrees of reflexivity, about how things are and why they are as they are.

There are a few more preliminaries to be borne in mind before the substantive theories on society, social change and health that are especially pertinent to the issues raised in this volume are broached (see Scambler, 2018, 2023). As the previous paragraphs indicate, (empirical) data do not speak for themselves, as is still sometimes either claimed or assumed. In the remarks that follow I deploy a number of rubrics: 'absence', 'explanatory focus', 'scope', 'going beyond is versus ought', 'philosophical grounding', 'fallibilism', and 'permeable boundaries'.

- *Absence*: the concept of absence is borrowed from the work of Roy Bhaskar which is explored later in this chapter, although it did not originate with him. Being, Bhaskar maintained, is but a ripple on the surface of the ocean of non-being. What he means is that what presently *is* comprises but one possibility among others too innumerable and varied to even envisage. These possibilities cover *what might have been* (as reflected in the predilection for 'what-if' histories) and *what might yet be*. The importance of this for social and sociological theory lies in its ramifications. It is only too easy to focus exclusively on a sociology of the present, or an historical sociology of how the present came to be. To do so is entirely legitimate, but it distracts attention from absence, that is, from a sociology of what might have been and what might yet be. I have suggested in fact that this is one facet of a 'taming' of the discipline (Scambler, 1996). I return to the salience of this in some detail in the concluding chapter of this book.

- *Explanatory focus*: as far as explanatory focus is concerned, I envisage sociology as the scientific study of society deploying mixed methods and committed to causal explanation. The cardinal sin of epidemiologically minded sociologists of health inequalities is that they treat prediction and explanation as two sides of the same coin: to be able to predict is to have explained. Prediction is important in its own right of course, notably in the context of urgent public health intervention (consider COVID); but reducing social reality to expedient chunks called 'variables' is every bit as troublesome as twinning prediction and explanation. But, as has become clear, multivariate or positivist research is nevertheless grist to the mill of sociological enquiry.

- *Scope*: scope here refers to sociology's reach from the micro-through the meso- to the macro-study of social phenomena. This implies a commitment to plural methodologies. Consider, for example, the governing decisions taken by UK's political elite. As should already be apparent, to fully appreciate and account for the sociological significance of these it is necessary to trespass beyond any personal talents and perspicacity leaders may or may not possess to consider the historically generated and socially and culturally structured constraints and opportunities that came their way *in the era of contemporary British rentier capitalism*. Political leaders' profiles can only be properly explicated in this context. The present accent on individuals and individualism is a key aspect of the near-ubiquitous ideology of neoliberalism that affords cover for asset managers and rentiers.

- *Beyond is and ought*: the philosopher David Hume's argument that what 'ought' to be the case cannot be inferred from what 'is' the case still attracts a considerable following; indeed, it is an uninterrogated premiss of much quantitative sociology, most obviously in health inequalities research. This is ironic in that we are typically *against* inequality. Inequality is almost invariably studied with a view to its effective reduction. As we shall see later in this chapter, accounts of 'false consciousness' are necessarily evaluative. Moreover, these evaluations are likely to be in terms of the ideological use of cultural resources by dominant vested interest groups to retain and spread their power and privileges. If a theory emerges that explains why false consciousness is necessary, then (i) a negative evaluation of the social relations that made that consciousness necessary can be immediately reached, and (ii) a positive evaluation of rationally planned attempts to remove the causes of false consciousness demand consent. But more than exposing false consciousness is involved. Consider the wage-form in capitalism. This cannot be explicated (that is, truthfully accounted for) in the absence of a critique of capitalism as a system of class exploitation: a scientific analysis is at one and the same time a political-ethical critique if the wage-form is a mechanism of alienation and exploitation. Propositions in sociology, if true, deliver moral obligations 'by force of logical necessity' (Scambler, 2018: 21).
- *Philosophical grounding*: there are no foundations of absolute certainty on which the edifice of sociological knowledge can be constructed, but this does not mean that there is no need to 'ground' our theories. To adapt an analogy from Karl Popper, while it is not necessary, indeed a mistake, to attempt to sink piles to support an oil rig to a final end point of rock, it remains essential that they are driven 'deep enough' to do the job. This is another point to be developed later.
- *Fallibilism*: any theory we construct, whether about the natural or social world, can turn out to be only partially true, as when Newtonian theory was overtaken by Einstein's, or just plain false. This is one of the lessons of the past. The implication is twofold: it reminds us never to rest content with what Thomas

Kuhn called 'normal science', or the theoretical status quo; and it encourages a mindset that affords full acknowledgement of the provisional nature of the explanatory theories that sociologists adduce.

• *Permeable boundaries*: any discipline is confined and limited in its reach and scope. This amounts to an invitation to interdisciplinarity. It will be apparent that this volume has already drawn on research from a range of different disciplines in considering phenomena such as population health and climate change. Sociology is not only charged with investigating an 'open society' – that is, one that no assembly of theories can 'wrap up' – but must be ready to learn from, be receptive to and accommodate theories and research from other disciplines.

What is left of Marx for the fractured society?

The works of Marx have to this point informed the discussion – for example, while ruminating on class and class conflict and world systems theory – without being intrusive. While this is not the place for a scholarly critique, it is important for the arguments of the remaining chapters that more is said on the contemporary pertinence of what Marx wrote a century and a half ago. In this chapter the focus will be on social and sociological theories that help account for the shape and form of contemporary societies. In the following chapter the focus will be on theories of transformative change. Marx baulked at the idea that he was a 'bourgeois' sociological theorist, but he has remained a vital catalyst for thinking about the nature of society into the 21st century. Moreover, the 'basics' of Marx's thinking have retained their thrust. After discussing Marx's writings, the attention turns, with equivalent brevity, to the contributions of Jurgen Habermas and Roy Bhaskar.

Rejecting Hegelian idealism, which exclusively inhabited the realm of ideas accessed through consciousness, Marx stressed that ideas and consciousness, alike, are part and parcel of material activity and interaction. It is not that ideas like those advanced in this slim volume cannot be debated, but rather that this presupposes a set of material conditions, for example 'academies' based on a separation of mental and physical labour. Only when a society has achieved an economic surplus over material necessity, releasing some of its members from the demands of productive labour, can such a debate occur. Marx then is interested in the material causes and conditions of thought itself. The assembly and institutionalisation of ideas (that is, culture) is for him rooted in labour, and therefore in exploitation. Capitalism, he argued, is characterised by a fundamental distinction between those who own capital, the *bourgeoisie*, and those who must sell their labour for wages, the *proletariat*. In a much-quoted passage from the *Communist Manifesto* he and Engels did not hold back:

> The bourgeoisie cannot exist without constantly revolutionising the instruments of production, and thereby the relations of production, and with them the whole relations of society. ... Constant revolutionising of production, uninterrupted disturbance of all social conditions, everlasting uncertainty and agitation distinguish the bourgeois epoch from all earlier ones. All fixed, fast-frozen relations, with their train of ancient and venerable prejudices and opinions, are swept away, all new-formed ones become antiquated before they can ossify. All that is solid melts into air, all that is holy is profaned, and man is at last compelled to face with sober senses, his real conditions of life, and his relations with his kind.

There is no doubt that passages like this retain their resonance in today's fractured societies, as do others in his family of interlinked theses. What we think and say, for Marx, is largely determined by what we do. In the social production of our lives we enter into relations of production that creep up on us unawares and are independent of our will. These relations correspond to stages of development of the forces of material production. He distinguishes between base and superstructure: all social and political forms, and all significant social change, have their roots in material production. Marx's point here is that in capitalism the base of social relations is unjust and contradictory, with the result that the superstructure of ideas functions politically to legitimate this ('the ideas of the ruling class are in every epoch the ruling ideas').

In this manner the ruling ideas constitute an ideology, that is, they amount to a view of the world that rationalises (bourgeois) vested interests.

Adam Smith had been aware of the predictable and inexorable polarisation of people in 'free-market capitalism', whereby the rich become richer and the poor poorer, and he commended ameliorative intervention. What Marx added was a theory of exploitation, crystallised in his theory of surplus value. This can be articulated via three claims that were relatively uncontroversial in Fordist industrial capitalism and are, arguably, still pertinent into financialised or rentier capitalism. These claims are that: (i) objects and services have a 'use value' and an 'exchange value'; (ii) what wage-labourers are paid to produce these objects and services is less than accrues to their capital-owning employers via their sale – that is, their exchange value – thereby generating a surplus for the latter; and (iii) wage-labourers therefore fund grandiose lifestyles for the bourgeoisie via exchange/surplus value to which they can themselves never aspire. Moreover, people come to see the exchange value of any particular object or service not as a product of labour, but as a naturally given and fixed property of the commodity. Commodities assume 'thing-like' relations with each other. What is social comes to be viewed as natural. 'Commodity fetishism', in short, disguises real social relations of production: they do not appear for what they are.

Capitalists pursue their profits through accumulation, but this can only be achieved at the expense of those who provide the labour power. Over time, *even if the income of the wage-labourer or worker increases as a concomitant of the rapid growth of capital*, at the same time a material and social chasm will open up between worker and capitalist, together with a general increase in the power of capital over labour and a greater dependence of labour on capital. This structural contradiction sits at the core of capitalism in all its guises. At this juncture, it only remains to say a word or two about alienation. Primarily in his earlier studies, Marx developed an account of worker estrangement or alienation under capitalism. He distinguished four types. First, workers are alienated from the product, over which they have neither ownership nor control. Second, they are alienated from the labour process, over which they have no say and which is experienced as a compulsory pursuit of extrinsic but not intrinsic worth. Third, they are alienated from their fellow workers, with whom they are essentially competing. And finally, they are alienated from 'what it is to be human' since any natural human belonging and solidarity is overcome by correlates of the relentless pursuit of profit.

All this understates the subtlety of Marx's work, most obviously in *Das Capital*. He was very aware, for example, that different capitalist societies had different class compositions. Nor, notwithstanding statements in the *Communist Manifesto*, did he in *Das Capital* dispute the emergence of new 'middling classes'. He was fully aware, in Evans' (2023: 144) words, that

> the concentration of capital requires increasing levels of oversight, a proliferation of management tiers, with the shift to global supply chains requiring complex logistics and legal and accounting roles, the necessary expansion of finance for the free circulation of capital globally, increased workers to promote the increased surplus product and so on.

But Marx did predict that *over time* starker polarisations between bourgeoise and proletariat would eventually occur; that these polarisations would ultimately unleash revolutionary proletarian impulses (the proletarian class 'in-itself' would mutate into a class 'for-itself'); and that these revolutions would, in turn, see a transition from capitalist to post-capitalist or communist societies. While he was in no sense an economic determinist, he was, in the event, over-optimistic. Historic state interventionism, culminating in postwar welfare statism, combined with the mushrooming of 'intermediary' middle classes, were key to dousing any revolutionary sparks, let alone wildfires.

If this briefest of explications of Marx's sociological insights and theories contains messages for the present, how to summarise? There are innumerable elaborations, developments and critiques of texts that have after all aged in a century and a half, both on the part of Marxists and non-Marxists. Interesting though this literature is, a scholarly and critical perusing of them is no part of the project this book represents. Neither the extent to which Marx was and/or is right nor the fidelity or otherwise of uses of his work are immediate concerns. These issues matter of course, but they can also deflect attention from matters of presence, *and absence*, pertaining to our contemporary human habitats. But there is a case for an addendum or two, the first of which elaborates on the discussion and conceptualisation of class that drew on the work of neo-Marxist Erik Ohlin Wright and was summarised in Chapter Four. Wright made a point of noting the existence of 'contradictory class locations', most notably in relation to the emerging and growing 'middle classes' that are obstinately intermediate between the bourgeoisie and proletariat. Wright argues that 'not all positions in the social structure can be seen as firmly rooted in a single class: some positions occupy objectively contradictory locations between classes' (cited in Evans, 2023). People can and do have contradictory needs and interests. Evans (2023: 39) captures Wright's stance in the following words:

> He argues that some people simply occupy the grey areas on the boundaries between classes and may therefore have elements of the interests (and ideologies) of both classes. Thus some people may occupy the border between the proletariat and the petty bourgeoise (for example, foremen), some between the petty bourgeoise and the bourgeoisie (technicians and managers) and so on. This is not so different to Marx's conception of the petty bourgeoisie as being 'cut up into two' and caught between the capitalist and the proletariat.

In other words, for Wright class boundaries possess a degree of permeability.

Evans goes on to develop this notion of the petty bourgeoisie in an interesting and relevant way. Conventionally, in Marxist and non-Marxist literatures alike, the petty bourgeoisie refers to those who owned their own means of production as small craftsmen and small farmers; these people comprised a class that occupied an 'interstitial' position in the class structure between the working class and the bourgeoisie. They were distinguished by their autonomy and social isolation, which set them apart from members of the proletariat who worked together collectively in large-scale production. Marx saw the petty bourgeoisie as a 'transitional class', predicting that it would be rendered largely redundant by large-scale manufacturing. But, Evans shows, this traditional or 'old' petty bourgeoisie has instead grown significantly and changed. It is no longer characterised by low technology and traditional work practices, though it remains socially isolated and exists in conditions of precarity.

Evans draws a distinction between the traditional or old petty bourgeoisie and what he calls the *new petty bourgeoisie*. The latter has mushroomed via deindustrialisation and the switch to services. Its members now tend to work in white-collar industries and are often 'educated' and culturally distinct from the old petty bourgeoisie. But while economically close to the proletariat because people do not own their own means of production, white-collar workers are socially and ideologically placed in the petty bourgeoisie because they inhabit a class which is fluid and, hence, often precarious, and has 'inculcated within it the same individualism, status anxiety and need for distinction as the petty bourgeoisie of old' (Evans, 2023: 309). Why does this matter? It does so because, insofar as Evans' refinement of Wright's analysis is warranted, this significantly expanded, or new, petty bourgeoisie has at various periods of history helped underpin neoliberalism and undermine collectivism. The left, Evans argues, must urgently come to terms, theoretically and politically, with this volatile class if it is to usher in significant or transformative social change. This is an issue that is directly confronted in Chapter Ten.

The second addendum arises out of the fact that in his later and largely unpublished writings Marx was giving serious consideration to environmental issues; and these writings warrant attention here. In his *Capital, Nature and the Unfinished Critique of Political Economy* and *Marx and the Anthropocene*, Kohei Saito's (2017, 2023) scholarly examination of these writings is a key source. His textual studies show that towards the end of his life Marx was actively researching the field of environmental challenges. He was examining the literatures on geology, botany and agricultural chemistry with a view to developing an analysis of the 'various practices of robbery closely tied to climate change, the exhaustion of natural resources (soil nutrients, fossil fuel and woods) as well as the extinction of species due to the capitalist system of industrial production' (Saito,

2023: 4). Saito notes the importance in Marx's theory of what John Bellamy Foster (2000) has termed a 'metabolic rift'. This notion of a metabolic rift opens up the possibility of extending Marx's critique of capitalism's destructive side to encompass contemporary as well as historical ecological matters such as global warming, soil erosion, aquaculture, the livestock business and the disruption of the nitrogen cycle. According to this reading, Marx's embryonic theory, which Foster relates to his early work on alienation, postulates an 'irreparable rift' or rupture in the metabolic interaction between humanity and the rest of nature that was initially a function of capitalist agricultural production and the escalating division between town and country. Metabolism is Marx's mature analysis of the alienation of nature. Far from neglecting the environment, the theory of metabolic rift detectable in Marx's writings enabled Marx to develop a critique of environmental degradation that anticipated much of present-day ecological thought. Unsurprisingly Marxist scholars have yet to reach a consensus on all this, and hindsight is a mixed blessing; but the door remains ajar for commentators inclined towards a neo-Marxist theory of an already-fractured 'world at risk' via climate change – among other threats – and at renewed peril in rentier capitalism. As we shall see in the penultimate chapter of this book, much present debate coalesces around the contentious concept of 'de-growth'.

The framework of Jurgen Habermas

Jurgen Habermas began his sociological career as a neo-Marxist critical theorist but has long since modified his thinking. His value at this point in this book lies in the framework he spelled out in detail in the two volumes of his *Theory of Communicative Action* (1984, 1987). I have argued in some detail elsewhere that it is a merit of his theorising that it allows for and encourages an interlinking of micro-, meso- and macro-sociological theories (Scambler, 2001, 2020). A core distinction in Habermas' work is that between 'system' and 'lifeworld'. It is a distinction that has a dual function. First, it characterises a worldwide tension in rentier capitalism; and second, it is a useful conceptual and heuristic device. The lifeworld for Habermas is the everyday world of sociability within which we interact and build relationships. These relations are typically rooted in trust and reciprocity, or what Habermas calls 'communicative action', namely, action oriented to consensus. People's use of language, Habermas argues, implies a common endeavour to attain consensus in a context in which all participants are free to contribute and have an equal chance of doing so. The use of language, in other words, presupposes a commitment to an 'ideal speech situation' in which discourse can realise its full potential. This, he insists, is a universal presupposition, free from any particular historical context. The idea of rationally motivated shared understanding – and rational motivation implies a total lack of compulsion or manipulation – is built into the very reproduction of social life. The symbolic reproduction of social life, it can be said, is founded on the counterfactual ideal of the ideal speech situation, which is characterised by 'communicative symmetry' and a compulsion-free consensus.

The lifeworld must be contrasted with the system. The system encompasses the economy and state and is characterised by 'strategic action', or action oriented to outcome. The modern, Western, post-Enlightenment world has seen a differentiation of both lifeworld and system into distinct spheres, as well as a discernible and profoundly significant 'decoupling' of lifeworld and system. Moreover, *the system has come to 'colonise' the lifeworld*. Habermas expounds on this claim as follows. He divides each of the lifeworld and the system into two sectors, as represented in Box 9.1.

Box 9.1: Lifeworld and system

LIFEWORLD	SYSTEM
(Communicative action)	(Strategic action)
Private sphere	**Economy**
(for example, household)	(for example, markets)
Steering media = COMMITMENT	Steering media = MONEY
Public sphere	**State**
(for example, mainstream media)	(for example, bureaucracy)
Steering media = INFLUENCE	Steering media = POWER

The private sector of the lifeworld, epitomised in the household, generates 'commitment'; and the public sector of the lifeworld, since Habermas was writing extended to the Internet and social media such as Twitter/X, Facebook, Instagram and so on, gives rise to 'influence'. The economic sector of the system encompasses a series of global markets and acts through its steering media of 'money', or capital. And the state sector of the system, featuring a long-armed legal and bureaucratic apparatus, is where 'power' derives and is exercised. I have paraphrased Habermas' point about colonisation as follows:

> the strategic, outcome-oriented system has, through its steering media of money and power, come progressively in modernity to impose itself on, even dictate to, the mundane communicative action, oriented to consensus, of the lifeworld. Commitment and influence have in the process become manipulated and perverted, or more bluntly, bought and regulated. (Scambler, 2020: 24)

It will be apparent from the substantive material accumulated in previous chapters that there is a strong prima facie case for deploying this Habermasian framework in this volume. Lifeworlds globally have been constrained and skewed by the unfolding of capitalism, and at an accelerating pace during post-1970s' financialised or rentier capitalism.

I mentioned earlier that it is a compelling property of Habermas' theorising that it allows for and exhorts linkages between macro-, meso- and micro-sociological theories. I have sought to illustrate elsewhere just how the macro-phenomena of lifeworld/system decoupling, and the subsequent colonising intrusions of the latter into the former, can play out in routine exchanges between doctors and patients (Scambler, 1987). Summarising here, Habermas shows how the taken-for-granted communicative ethos can be subverted by strategic action. He focuses first on the notion of 'open strategic action', which occurs when money and/or power are conspicuously and tellingly on display to demand acquiescence and consent. 'Concealed strategic action' can take one of two forms: (i) 'distorted communication', or manipulation, takes place when one party to an exchange is being strategic and hides or disguises this from the other; 'systematically distorted communication' occurs when both parties to an exchange are acting in good faith but one party is acting strategically, for example, according to an agenda about which he or she is unaware or non-reflexive. Using these concepts, Habermas provides for an examination of the impact of macro-structural and social and cultural change on routine everyday encounters in the lifeworld via what he – rather strangely – calls a 're-feudalised' public sphere of the lifeworld.

Notwithstanding his own self-distancing from Marx, the suitability of Habermas' theoretical framework to accommodate the neo-Marxist perspective on health and health care developed in this book might be illustrated in two ways. The first relates to the core mechanism introduced, that of the class/command dynamic: it is a hard core of transnational and nomadic financiers, CEOs and their allies that have come increasingly to lobby and 'buy' sufficient power from the elite politicians in nation states to steer policies their way, that is, to promote company and personal capital accumulation. This dynamic, it has been noted, helps underpin and fuel a range of other dynamics with high salience for the contemporary UK and further afield, namely, the stigma/deviance, insider/outsider, elite/mass and party/populist dynamics. Insofar as the prepotent class/command dynamic, together with its variable causal input into the other dynamics, can be interpreted as systemic and strategic intrusions into the lifeworld via the steering media of money plus power, they can be represented as forms of lifeworld colonisation. In other words, they involve a usurpation, warping and perversion of the communicative action that is the template of ordinary everyday discourse. At this point Habermas' analysis kicks in again. Using his terminology, it can be said that the public sphere of the lifeworld, which he rightly saw as deeply contaminated by the mass media of late Fordist/Welfare capitalism, is now open to further strategic confounding via the Internet and social media outlets born of late financial/rentier capitalism. The public sphere, seat of influence, is much changed. Class/command entryism has not only refined the long-established public school/Oxford University pathway into the traditional mass media but is ramping up the funding and mass media exposure of a series of so-called think tanks that can be relied on to toe and evangelise around the ideological line. Box 9.2 gives a summary of the role of dark money, dirty politics and think tanks currently operating in the UK. The term 'dark money' is a familiar one in US politics and refers to those monies clandestinely invested to warp democratic processes such as elections. Dark money disseminates ideology at the expense of knowledge via the medium of think tanks.

Box 9.2: Leading think tanks in the UK

Some of the most influential think tanks are listed here, together with (i) their political orientation, and (ii) their degree of transparency re: their funders. I have taken as a measure of transparency a rating from A (totally open) to E (totally closed) deployed by the 'UK Campaign for Think Tank Transparency'. A indicates that the think tank is open about its income, and declares the amounts given. E indicates that the think tank fails all these tests.

Adam Smith Institute (ASI)
The prime focus of the ASI is the introduction of free-market policies. (E)
Centre for Policy Studies (CPS)
Founded by Thatcher in 1974, the CPS aims to promote free-market policies and limit the role of the state. (E)
Centre for Social Justice (CSJ)
Established by Iain Duncan Smith in 2004 to seek solutions to social breakdown and poverty, with a focus on the voluntary sector combatting poverty. (D)
Demos
Founded in 1993, Demos is a cross-party think tank interested in welfare and public services, education, citizenship and social media. (B)
Fabian Society
Founded in 1884 and affiliated to the Labour Party, the Fabian Society is a major left-of-centre think tank. (A)
Institute for Economic Affairs (IEA)
One of the oldest in the UK, the IEA is a high-profile right-wing think tank that promotes free-market solutions to a wide range of social and economic issues. (E)

High Pay Centre (HPC)

Set up to monitor top levels of pay. (A)

Institute for Fiscal Studies (IFS)

Established to provide independent research on economic and fiscal policy. (A)

Institute for Public Policy Research (IPPR)

Was formed following Labour's 1987 election defeat, aiming to invigorate left-wing thinking. (B)

The Legatum Institute

Set up as an international, right-of-centre liberal think tank focused on revitalising capitalism and democracy. (C)

New Economics Foundation (NEF)

An independent left-of-centre 'think and do' think tank that aims to promote alternative economic models, focusing also on social justice and environmental issues. (A)

Policy Exchange

A right-wing small-government think tank that conducts research into poverty and social mobility, public services and economic issues. (E)

Reform

An independent right-of-centre think tank that seeks to set out a way to lower public spending and increase prosperity. (C)

Resolution Foundation

Founded in 2005 to produce high-quality research and raise the profile of the challenges facing those on low to middle incomes and to develop policy solutions. (B)

Social Market Foundation (SMF)

The SMF is an independent, liberal think tank that aims to combine market economics with social justice. (B)

Tax Justice Network

Launched in 2003 as an independent, left-of-centre and 'activist' think tank to push for 'justice' and systematic change in relation to tax, tax havens and financial globalisation. (A)

TaxPayers' Alliance (TPA)

A right-wing think tank established in 2004 to campaign for lower taxation and for reducing public expenditure. (E)

Source: Adapted from Scambler (2020)

This list comprises the main, 'loudest' and most influential think tanks. It should be added that the mainstream media in the UK have long since abandoned scholarly 'academic' expertise in favour of representatives from think tanks. This being the case, the – often ideological – allegiances of these spokespersons are a matter of significant import: who is paying them what, and in whose interests? Currently right-wing think tanks are gaining disproportionate exposure. Geographer Tom Slater (2014) has shown in detail how one think tank, the CSJ associated with Iain Duncan Smith (architect of Universal Credit), has invoked a litany of social pathologies (family breakdown, worklessness, antisocial behaviour, personal irresponsibility, out-of-wedlock childbirth, dependency) to 'manufacture ignorance' and rationalise welfare reform (that is, benefit cuts). Dark money and secretively funded right-wing think tanks are devices permitting hard core capital monopolists to make their purchase of policies conducive to the further accumulation of capital from the state's power elite acceptable to the public. What this does is further expose the deep underlying structures and relations of class and class conflict: denial of class conflict is itself a manifestation of that conflict (Scambler, 2020: 83).

The class/command dynamic is also infiltrating and endeavouring to bend digital media to its own ideological – neoliberal – ends (Kuper, 2022). Much political rhetoric can be defined in terms of distorted communication, or manipulation. Using the concept of John Austin (1962), such rhetoric can be described as 'performative': in short, its very purpose is to have a particular – ideological – effect on audiences. This is not of course to deny the extent to which the lifeworld is colonised more indirectly in the form of systematically distorted communication. The extent to which those I have identified as 'greedy bastards', namely, the fraction of the 1 per cent and their allies who surf extant social structures to their advantage, actually come to believe that they are acting in the interests of the population as a whole is a moot point.

Habermas also devotes considerable attention to the project of 'lifeworld rationalisation'. Unlike one of his mentors, Max Weber, he neither sees the colonisation of the lifeworld by the system as historically inevitable, nor is he as pessimistic about the possibilities for future lifeworld rationalisation or resistance. But this is a theme to be revisited in far more detail in the next chapter. Now is an opportune time to turn to another philosopher and social theorist who sought to develop Marx's approach to capitalism.

Roy Bhaskar's underlabouring philosophy of critical realism

Whereas Jurgen Habermas was a social theorist first and foremost, Roy Bhaskar's (1975, 1989) overriding commitment was to philosophy. His ambitious intent was to provide Marxist analysis with a better philosophical grounding as well as to extend its scope and reach. Once again, I must be brief (for fuller accounts see Scambler, 2018, 2023). Too many philosophers past and present, Bhaskar argues, have committed the 'epistemic fallacy': they have reduced what 'is' to what we do and can 'know' of what is. In philosophical parlance they have reduced ontology (the study of being) to epistemology (the study of knowledge). He commends a 'realist ontology'. In short, the planet we currently inhabit, together with a range of non-human species of fauna and flora, would continue to exist even if we humans managed to accomplish our own extinction, for example via climate or thermonuclear catastrophe. Moreover, reality – the 'real' – is multi-layered or 'stratified'. It is causal interaction at 'lower strata or levels' (the objects of interest to physicists, for example) that gives rise to 'higher strata or levels' (the objects of interest to the likes of life scientists, psychologists and sociologists). The latter 'emerge from' but are not 'reducible to' the former.

This schema allows for a distinctively sociological contribution to the study of health and health care while recognising the salience of 'interdisciplinarity'. As far as methodology is concerned, critical realists typically argue for a version of 'critical naturalism'. This accepts both a degree of unity across the natural, life and social sciences *and* that sociologists cannot conduct their studies under laboratory conditions. The phenomena of interest to sociologists exist in an 'open system'. The objects of sociological knowledge – social structures and relations – 'are internally rather than externally related, quite unlike the relations between the socially generated natural sciences and their *non-social* objects of knowledge' (Creaven, 2007: 9). Although the methods of natural and social scientists are certainly not identical, they share the same goal, namely, the pursuit of causal explanations for phenomena of concern to them.

For Bhaskar, the pursuit in which natural and social scientists are engaged is for those 'real' mechanisms that must exist for us to experience events as we do. In sociology attention switches from the flux of events (constant or otherwise) and towards the causal mechanisms, social structures and relations that deliver them. These mechanisms are 'intransitive', that is, they exist whether or not they are detected. It is not possible to simply map the effects of mechanisms at the level of events and our perceptions of them: such is the nature of an open system. This is because mechanisms act 'transfactually'. Once set in motion, or triggered, they continue to exert an influence even if other countervailing mechanisms neutralise this influence (the focus in this volume has been on social class as the key capitalist mechanism, but clearly there are contexts in which this mechanism is neutralised by countervailing mechanisms such as gender and race). The notion of 'tendencies' derived from Marxist economics has been used in this connection. Thus, the mechanisms that combine to issue in a tendency for the rate of profit to decline act transfactually; that is, they remain active even when empirically the rate of profit is rising. Their transfactuality is due to the operating of other mechanisms – for example, technological advances – acting in a countervailing manner. Beneath-the-surface class and command structures or relations, qua causal mechanisms, can and often do resist easy on-the-surface detection, in part because of countervailing mechanisms.

Bhaskar sees ontology as 'transformational' as well as stratified. He advances what he calls a 'transformational model of social action'. He intends this to supersede rival accounts of agency and structure. Agents do not create or produce structures *ab initio*, but rather *re*create, *re*produce and/or transform them into a set of pre-existing structures. The total ensemble of structures comprises/is society. He offers this oft-quoted summary in the following words:

> People do not create society. For it always pre-exists
> them and is a necessary condition for their activity.

Rather society must be regarded as an ensemble of structures, practices and conventions which individuals reproduce and transform, but would not exist unless they did so. Society does not exist independently of human activity (the error of reification). But it is not the product of it (the error of voluntarism). (Bhaskar, 1987: 129)

Sean Creaven (2007: 8) elaborates on this statement by referring once more to ontological stratification. Causal mechanisms, he reminds us, travel both 'upstream' (from lower to higher strata) or 'downstream' (from higher to lower strata):

At the same time as humanity's species being and attendant powers and capacities are transmitted 'upstream' into social interaction and socio-cultural relations (supplying the power which energises the social system, constraining and enabling social-cultural production and reproduction, and providing a certain impetus towards the universal articulation of particular kinds of cultural norms or principles), structural-cultural and agential conditioning are transmitted 'downstream' to human persons (investing in them specific social interests and capacities, shaping unconsciously much of their psychological and spiritual makeup, and furnishing them with the cultural resources to construct personal and social identities for themselves).

It is sufficient to note at this point that for all that Bhaskar's basic critical realism raises important philosophical issues that cannot be properly addressed here, I hope enough has been said to commend it to people interested in multi- and interdisciplinary orientations to individual, social and global health.

Before drawing together the web of rather abstruse threads in this chapter, a few more points arising from Bhaskar's critical realism warrant a mention. The first dips into his later or 'dialectical' critical realism and briefly revisits the idea of absence introduced at the beginning of this chapter. For

Bhaskar, absence or non-being is ontologically prior to presence or being. If, following Hegel, absence/non-being were to be entirely cancelled out by presence/being, the dialectic would cease, and along with it, evolution, emergence and change itself, leaving us with a Hegelian 'closed totality'. It is of the essence of dialectic that real absence or negativity energises the struggle for presence or positivity. It is in this context that Bhaskar's 'four planar' theory should be understood. This suggests that the dialectical interaction of agents with structural properties and/or practices can be considered on four analytically distinct planes. These are: *material transactions with nature* (that is, cooperative labour to produce subsistence); *social relations between agents* (as incumbents of structured 'positions' and 'practices' of the social system), *interpersonal relations* (interactions between individuals as subjects rather than as agents of positions and institutional roles); and *intra-subjective relations* (internal relations of the subject, such as the self-construction of personal and cultural identities) (Creaven, 2007: 31). It is axiomatic that recognition and analysis across this quartet of planes are both highly pertinent to any credible explanatory (and emancipatory) account of people confronted with today's collocation of and threats to health and wellbeing.

Among many other contributions to critical realism, Margaret Archer (2007) has enhanced the analysis of the fourth of Bhaskar's quartet of planes, intra-subjective relations, by writing of 'internal conversations'. These are conversations we all have – with ourselves – that constitute an important form of personal reflexivity as well as mediating the effects of structure on agency. We constantly deliberate about ourselves in relation to the social situations we face, she argues,

> certainly fallibly, certainly incompletely and necessarily under our own descriptions, because that is the only way we can know anything. To consider that human reflexivity plays a role of mediation also means entertaining the fact that we are dealing with two ontologies: the objective pertaining to social emergent properties and the subjective pertaining to agential emergent properties. (Archer, 2007: 42)

It follows that subjectivity is not only real but irreducible; *and that it possesses causal efficacy.*

A final point on Bhaskar concerns his distinction between 'power 1' and 'power 2' relations. As is the case with society, individuals are seen as stratified and relational entities. Power 1 relations refer to the transformative capacity intrinsic to the concept of agency as such. Power 2 relations involve a more sociological notion of power, denoting social relations that govern the distribution of material goods, political and military authority, and social and cultural stratification. Power 2 relations, in other words, are those that enable agents to defend their sectoral advantages by prevailing against the covert wishes and/or the real interests of others. Bhaskar insists that power is enabling and empowering and repressive. But the relevance here of power 2 relations is that 'they organise or structure the capacity of human agents to exercise transformative power over their conditions of existence, and so restrict the autonomy and free-flourishing of people subject to their governance' (Creaven, 2007: 32).

Tying together a few theoretical threads

Marx's theories clearly require amendment but not, in my view, abandonment. Any viable sociological analysis of contemporary globalised rentier capitalism should begin with Marx. This volume might therefore be classified as neo-Marxist. The UK in the 21st century remains a society divided and conflicted above all by social class. Marxian notions of class-based conditions, privileges and opportunities, as well as of sites of struggle, exploitation and alienation live on. For all that subjective senses of identity have become heavily coloured by cultural shifts centred on what has here been called cultural relativisation, meaning that any transition from class in-itself to class for-itself has grown complex, objective class has become more salient and intrusive in people's lives than was the case in postwar late Fordist/welfare state capitalism.

Despite Habermas removing himself from the Marxist fold, his theories of the modern decoupling of lifeworld and system and of communicative versus strategic action offer a useful framework for reformulating and repackaging Marx's bold if partially time-bound 19th-century theories. A credible neo-Marxist orientation to rentier capitalism can be recast as a distinctive type of lifeworld colonisation, whereby the economy and state's steering media of money and power, combined in the class/command dynamic, have penetrated close to the heart of the lifeworld, aided by what Habermas called the 're-feudalisation' of the public sphere but what might better be interpreted as the deployment of capital to underline and extend the ubiquity and influence of the ideology of neoliberalism via the mass and increasingly digital media. It might be protested that Habermas called on Weber and others as well as Marx when explicating his theory of lifeworld colonisation, but this is not to negate the substantial Marxian input into his theories.

If Habermas offers an alternative way of conceptualising and framing the emergence of contemporary capitalist ways of living in the UK and elsewhere, Bhaskar's explicitly neo-Marxist contribution is both to add a lively family of overlapping concepts and to delve more deeply into the philosophical grounding of sociological theorising and practice. In the closing chapter, which addresses rival agendas for the practice of sociology and makes a case for fortifying sociology's weak commitment to foresight and action sociology, I will outline and elaborate on Bhaskar's defence and advocacy of the rational or 'logical' goal of the universal free flourishing of all for all. But I hope it will already be apparent that the innovative conceptual apparatus offered up by Bhaskar's basic and dialectical critical realism has much to offer. The ontological priority of absence – of what might have been and might yet be – prises open options for analyses spanning his four planar arenas for study in what must always remain an open society. This is highly significant in relation to the necessarily interdisciplinary examination of health, health care and wellbeing in a strategic and imperial/colonising and still Occidental-run global system faced with a new 'world at risk'. Bhaskar's explication of agency/ structure/culture and powers 1 and 2 afford alternate ways of characterising and representing Marxian exploitation and a Habermasian system colonisation of the lifeworld. In the next chapter theories of transformative social change are adjudicated, together with the 'obstacles' they must circumvent.

TEN

A theoretical framework for achieving the healthy society

The focus of this book is necessarily as much on the obstacles to accomplishing health-bestowing change as it is on characterising and accounting for why such change is vital. And the canvas has, again necessarily, been large. As was suggested in the Introduction, my principal grouse against much sociological research on health inequalities, and much of the literature on policy recommendations too, is that they barely mention, or even ignore, social class and other beneath-the-surface or structural causal mechanisms and are, as a result, unrealistic and merely aspirational. The agendas of experts such as Michael Marmot are, of course, epidemiological rather than sociological. In our various personal and friendly exchanges, he has stressed that his concern is to provide the scientific evidence on health inequalities and to push for relevant policy reforms to secure their reduction. This is the commendable 'realism 1' of the insider. But health inequalities are currently widening in our fractured society and have been hit hard post-2010 by political austerity and COVID. An alternative approach is via the sociologist as outsider, and this is the one favoured here: my alternative 'realism 2' draws on the theories of Marx, Habermas and Bhaskar. And to reiterate, an immediate and pressing concern is why, despite their best-efforts, Marmot and his colleagues have *not* inspired effective policy change. Another conspicuous theme has been that health inequalities in the UK can *and should* no longer: (i) be broached in isolation from global health inequalities, and (ii) be divorced from pressing and ubiquitous risks, typically exported from the high-income core countries of the Global North to the low-income peripheral countries of the Global South, such as climate change and conventional and conceivably nuclear warfare and their sequelae.

Using an implicitly critical realist frame, it has been asked what social structures *must* exist for empirical studies of material, social and health inequalities to deliver the findings they have. Given the nature of the open society and the unavailability of experimental 'closures', sociologists have typically to rely on what Bhaskar calls 'retroductive inferences' from the 'demi-regularities' deriving from quantitative research, or what he calls 'abductive inferences' from qualitative or ethnographic research. There is, for example, a mass of quasi-epidemiological sociological research on health inequalities in the UK and elsewhere using proxies for social class like NS-SEC (see Introduction). Such findings, like those from a sparser range of more sociological endeavours engaging more intimate qualitative methods, are grist to the sociological mill. In combination, it has been maintained throughout this volume, they confirm that social class qua social structure *must* exist for the research to have come up with the consistent findings it has. So, to extend the analysis here, neo-Marxist explanatory theories come into play insofar as they provide credible theories around social class as 'a' – I would maintain 'the' – key or driving causal mechanism behind the complex *chain of mechanisms* that results in obstinately durable inequalities through capitalism. This chain of mechanisms, it was earlier suggested, might be interpreted in terms of the variable strength of a series of asset flows (biological, psychological, social, cultural, spatial, symbolic and material) known to impact on health and longevity. These asset flows were defined as the media of enactment of class relations on health. It is a notion that has of course to be adapted from society to society in a complex, dynamic and ever-changing world.

It follows from this line of argument that it is insufficient merely to give a passing mention to social structures such as class, gender, race and so on in the concluding paragraphs of scholarly papers on social, material, cultural and health inequalities. Bluntly put, that is a cop out. A by-product of this is the over-privileging of (insider) 'realism 1' over (outside) 'realism 2'. And there are temptations for academics to do precisely this in increasingly competitive and neoliberal academic environments in which attaining research funding and publishing in high-impact journals are crucial. I return to this matter in the final chapter. There are two points to stress now. It should be readily apparent by now, first, that class relations in the form of the nomadic transnational capital monopolists are causally responsible not just for underpinning, perpetuating and increasing inequality in affluent countries such as the UK, but worldwide. This influence is exposed too in recent research on climate change (for example, lobbying for fossil fuels) and armed conflict (for example, selling arms to all-comers). The second is that just as structural class relations are causally paramount for generating social and health inequalities, *so they are causally paramount both in diverting academic and public attention from this and in scuppering policy initiatives to affect transformational structural change.*

It is this latter point that provides the focus of the present chapter. Indeed, the book as a whole is as much about the 'obstacles' to accomplishing significant structural, cultural and agential change as it is about the need to do so. The discussion commences with a few paragraphs on mobilising for change.

Abrams' affinity-convergence model of spontaneous mass mobilisation

As Habermas moved away from the influence of Marx, he came to attribute less salience to social class and more to alternative drivers of change. His attention, and attention within European-then-American sociology generally, switched especially to the potentials contained in 'new social movements' (Habermas focused on feminism). The role of culture assumed more prominence and that of social class less in discussions of individual and collective protest and emancipation as late Fordist/welfare capitalism transmuted into finance/rentier capitalism and the class composition and divisions of societies like Britain grew less conspicuous and clear-cut. A substantial literature on factors affecting popular mobilisation accumulated. Often sociologists and social psychologists drew on classical theories of relative deprivation or collective behaviour to this end. In his excellent *The Rise of the Masses*, Benjamin Abrams (2023) offers summary statements. In *Why Men Rebel*, Ted Gurr (1970) used the concept of relative deprivation to better understand the emergence of social protests and rebellions. He commended refining enquiries to three areas: 'popular discontent' (relative deprivation); 'people's justifications or beliefs about the justifiability and utility of political action'; and 'the balance between discontented people's capacity to act – that is, the ways in which they are organised – and the government's capacity to repress or channel their anger' (see Abrams, 2023: 16). Of this triad, Gurr attributed most significance to relative deprivation, or the shortfall between the standard of living people expect from the social order and that which it provides for them. This discrepancy, he argued, resulted in a perception of injustice among groups which served to underpin participation in collective action.

Accounts drawing on the notion of collective behaviour started from a different standpoint. Collective behaviour occurs, its advocates contended, in unstructured conditions, or when established organisations have either lost their grip or no longer exist. The emphasis here was on spontaneous action. Abrams (2023: 17) writes:

> Theorists also posited that there might be some form of dispositional vulnerability to participation in a social movement, which was suggested to arise from emotional, cognitive, or personality traits, such as a sense of 'heightened frustration ... relative deprivation, alienation, (and) spoiled or stigmatised identities', as well as, in the case of more charismatic causes, an authoritarian personality. More than this, these theories even indicated that otherwise unconnected individuals' psychological and social traits could underpin spontaneous participation in collective behaviour without, or even in defiance of, formal organisation.

Abrams' interest in such theorising arises out of his own research on spontaneous mass mobilisation, and its relevance here is that he formulates an expedient conceptual framework, or model, for appraising the potential for collective mobilisations to effect structural change conducive for health and wellbeing nationally and further afield. It is a model into which the causal power of class will, in due course, be reintroduced.

Spontaneous mass mobilisation occurs, according to Abrams, when large numbers of people come together to partake in contentious politics without reliance on social movement organisations and their networks. His project is to lay out a comprehensive theoretical framework for this phenomenon. He calls his theory *affinity-convergence theory*: 'where sufficient affinity for a cause exists among a large group of people in society *and* convergence conditions arise or are effected in that same society, the conditions for spontaneous mass mobilisation are satisfied' (Abrams, 2023: 5). On many occasions mass mobilisation involves organisational forces, but not always. Sometimes people mobilise and organised forces are caught by surprise: Abrams suggests this occurred in relation to the uprising in Egypt, the Occupy Movement in New York, the Black Lives reaction to police brutality in the US and, historically, the French Revolution (his research focused on this quartet). Affinity-convergence theory purports to analyse and dissect the phenomenon of spontaneous mass mobilisation, first by addressing the issue of predisposition to participate in a cause (affinity), then by tackling the issue of how shifts in social conditions can encourage people to act on these predispositions (convergence).

Abrams offers typologies of both psychological and social affinities. It will be sufficient here merely to list these to give a sense of the comprehensiveness of his model. His analysis of psychological affinities focuses on 'identity', 'perceived injustice', 'attitudes', 'interests' and 'needs'. Social affinities are clustered under the following rubrics: 'patterns of activity', 'social status', 'resources' and 'obligations'. While Abrams convincingly demonstrates the causal salience of each of these, our most pressing concern here is on aspects of the sociology of convergence. He breaks convergence down into three subtypes. It can, first, be *opportune*. This can make participation in a cause more likely to yield positive results and less likely to inflict costs. Examples might include a collapse in state repression, an emergent conviction that change is achievable, or even a particular location with strategic or protective properties (as with the Occupy Movement's taking over of New York's Zuccotti Park). Second, convergence can be *exceptional*. This comes about when participation is facilitated for those with affinity to a cause. This might occur, for example, when long-established social rules and norms give way and an anomic situation ensues, bringing in its wake a generalised sense of permissiveness. And Abram's third subtype is when convergence becomes *paramount*. This is when ordinary incentive structures are overcome or overridden. 'This can take the form of a particular situation that made participation more palatable on the basis of different structural incentives, or a cognitive frame highlighting the importance of participation in a "historical moment" or in response to a moral shock' (Abrams, 2023: 45). This conceptualisation of spontaneous mobilisation will be utilised in the discussion of the state of play and the prospects of transformative social change in 21st-century Britain.

Social preconditions for transformative change

It is neither necessary to scorn nor altogether to dismiss the multiple attempts to reform capitalism to make it less predatory and more open to material and social inclusion. But its predatory characteristics have generally reasserted themselves, as is the case in the present phase of financialised or rentier capitalism. And it has been an omnipresent theme of this book that stratification by social class is of the essence of capitalism, and that structural class relations issue in class struggles over the strength of flow of those assets that hold the promise of a decent life. It has been argued too that these same asset flows are critical for health status and longevity. In as far as there are discernible structural powers behind health intra- and international inequalities – as I have contended, most often attributable to the class/command and related dynamics – then it is apparent that transformative change will require collective action beyond Karl Popper's piecemeal social engineering. And given the conspicuous absence of collective agents organised sufficiently to address this 'structural deficit', Abrams' thesis on spontaneous mass mobilisation is prescient.

This discourse cuts to the chase with regard to many extant sociologies of health inequalities. Without underplaying, let alone undermining, the sterling labours and policy recommendations of Marmot and his associates at the World Health Organization

(WHO) as well as colleagues in policy sociology, it is undeniable that they have sowed multiple seeds on stony ground. So how might the structural substrates of societies like Britain be challenged? Erik Ohlin Wright (2019) distinguishes several different strategies, or 'strategic logics'. *Smashing capitalism* is the uncompromising term he uses to refer to the classic strategic logic of the revolutionary and is associated with Marx, Lenin, Gramsci and others. Wright immediately acknowledges that this would be a 'daunting task'. Moreover, the results of revolutionary seizures of power in the 20th century 'were never the creation of a democratic, egalitarian, emancipatory alternative to capitalism' (Wright, 2019: 40). While revolutions in the name of socialism and communism did demonstrate that it was possible 'to build *a* new world from the ashes of the old', and although the material lives of most people may have been improved for a time, they did not deliver the kind of new world envisioned in revolutionary blueprints or thinking. System-level rupture, Wright concludes, does not work.

The second strategic logic is that of *dismantling capitalism*. Rejecting the notion of a revolutionary rupture, its advocates argued for an extended period in which both capitalist and socialist relations coexist in a mixed economy: 'There would be private capitalist banks alongside state-run banks; private capitalist firms alongside state enterprises, especially in transportation, utilities, health care, and certain branches of heavy industry; there would be capitalist labour markets alongside state employment; state-directed planning for allocations of investment alongside private profit-maximising investment' (Wright, 2016: 43). In this scenario there would be no simple moment of rupture but rather a gradual dismantling of capitalism and construction of alternative institutions, all overseen by the state. A precondition of such a transition would be a stable electoral democracy and a socialist party with sufficient mass support to underwrite a sustained period in office. There was much talk of the potential for a mixed economy and state-directed reform during Attlee's time in office in the UK (1945–51), but disillusionment with a reformist path to socialism was to set in shortly after.

Taming capitalism is Wright's third strategy. Unlike both smashing and dismantling capitalism, both of which, for all their differences over means to ends, can be said to have revolutionary agendas geared to replacing capitalism with a fundamentally different kind of economic structure, taming capitalism is oriented to neutralising capitalism's harms. Capitalism, when left to its own devices, 'creates great harms' (as we have seen throughout this short volume).

> It generates levels of inequality that are destructive to social cohesion; it destroys traditional jobs and leaves people to fend for themselves; it creates uncertainty and risk in the lives of individuals and whole communities; it harms the environment. These are all consequences of the inherent dynamics of a capitalist economy. (Wright, 2019: 45)

But capitalism can be tamed by well-crafted state policies oriented to counteract its most disruptive symptoms. This requires popular mobilisation and political will: sometimes, Wright writes in summarising this logic, neutralising the symptoms of capitalism is preferable to trying to remove the underlying cause.

The next strategic logic to be considered is *resisting capitalism*. This denotes anti-capitalist struggles that oppose capitalism from outside the state. It may involve influencing the state or blocking state actions, but it does not involve exercising state power. The focus here is on impacting the behaviour of capitalists and political elites through protests and other types of resistance outside of the state. It may not be possible to transform capitalism, but citizens can defend themselves from its harms by 'causing trouble, protesting and raising the costs to elites of their actions'. Grassroots activism in its various guises often falls into this category (for example, 'Just Stop Oil'). Another basic form of resisting capitalism is by citizens withholding their maximum effort and diligence.

Finally, Wright introduces and describes the strategic logic of *escaping capitalism*. Capitalism, its proponents contend, is too powerful a system to destroy, let alone dismantle and replace. The powers that be are simply too strong. The optimal strategy is, therefore, for people to 'remove themselves' from its orbit, for example by creating their own micro-alternatives within which they can live and flourish. Workers' cooperatives might furnish examples here, as do various 'drop out' – note the hippie motto of the 1960s' America, 'turn on, tune in, drop out' – or utopian communities. In contemporary Western societies escape often denotes an individualistic lifestyle strategy. Wright is wary of dismissing the strategic logic of escaping capitalism as a form of anti-capitalism on the grounds that it has in the past, and may yet, provided models for more collective, egalitarian and democratic ways of living (for example, cooperatives).

Wright pulls these threads together via the metaphor of a game. Smashing capitalism directs its aim at the game itself, at 'transcending structures'. Dismantling capitalism also aims at transcending structures, but by challenging and changing the rules of the game. Taming capitalism aims at 'neutralising harms' by altering the rules of the game. Resisting capitalism also has in its sights the neutralising of harms, but by concentrating on moves in the game. Finally, escaping capitalism aims at transcending structures, in this case also via a focus on moves in the game. It is a neat summary. But what significance does it have for us here? It has made clear that what is required to enhance greater equality of health and health care in the UK is transcending structures rather than neutralising harms. Moreover, such is the intimate, dialectical and fraught character of globalisation in the 21st century that it is not possible for an isolated and insulated UK to go it alone. And, critically, the external threats to the UK in the form of climate change and, conceivably, conventional-to-nuclear warfare (though likely motivated further afield) also tie the UK to events elsewhere.

Wright goes on to argue that three concepts are vital for grasping behaviours around transformative change: 'identities', 'interests' and 'values':

• *Identities*: people have multiple identities, and the subjective salience of any of them is dependent on context. But identities are not simply descriptive: they are intimately linked to social relations and power. They may be imposed and cultivated. They play a crucial role in the formation of 'collective actors'. Strong shared identities can increase trust and predictability among potential participants in collective action and facilitate the formation of durable collective actors. Especially salient for the formation of 'emancipatory collective actors' are identities rooted in those forms of socially imposed inequality and domination leading to 'real harms' (for example, disrespect, deprivations, disempowerment, bodily insecurity and abuse). Identities change over time. Moreover, identities cultivated within social movements can lead to deep connections with other collective actors engaged in struggles (for example, political parties, social movement organisations, labour unions).

- *Interests*: identities, Wright contends, are subjectively salient classifications of persons. Interests, on the other hand, refer to things that would improve a person's life along some dimension important to that person. Interests are anchored in the solutions to the problems people encounter in their lives; identities are anchored in the lived experiences generated in part by those problems. People can be mistaken about their interests, hence the notion of 'false consciousness'. Life is complex, as are people's identities, so people can have interests which are in tension, and even incompatible (for example, religious and sexual). They also have short- and long-term interests.

- *Values*: people act in a meaningful world, so values are involved (that is, beliefs about what is good and right). Values, Wright observes, have a fraught relationship to interests. For example, when political conservatives defend tax cuts for the rich by insisting that through increasing investment and thus economic growth this is the best way to help the poor (that is, trickle-down economics), they are invoking a general social value: poverty is a bad thing and a good society is one in which the lives of the least advantaged improve over time. Most people would agree with this affirmation of values. *If* it were true that cutting taxes for the rich was the best way to help the poor, this would be a powerful reason to support such policies. Of course, this view of tax cuts is an ideological rationalisation of the interests of the rich. Values can be powerful sources of motivation, and a robust source of identity. They can also fuel emancipatory thinking and action.

Drawing on this triad, Wright develops his theme. Accepting that identities, interests and values do not in and of themselves promise the formation of collective actors, he puts forward three principal challenges to the process of constructing collective actors capable of sustained political action. The first challenge is to *overcome privatised lives*. There is typically a gulf between private lives and public involvement. The second involves *building class solidarity within complex, fragmented class structures*. There is a need to forge strong working-class identities: the identity-interests of workers would then form the core of progressive politics that embraced the more universal interests linked to values of equality, democracy and solidarity. As things stand in 21st-century US and UK, however, it is necessary to navigate a multiplicity of intersecting identities that share common underlying emancipatory values but nevertheless have distinct identity-interests. A major threat here is right-wing populism, which is mobilising people on the basis of interests tied to exclusionary identities (for example, around race). Wright's third challenge involves *forging an anti-capitalist politics in the presence of diverse, competing non-class-based forms of identity*. Effective, politically organised collective action is essential for eroding capitalism. Pressing obstacles are people's privatised lives, the fragmental class structure and competing identities. Pulling these assorted threads together, Wright emphasises that values such as equality/fairness, democracy/freedom and community/ solidarity should remain at the centre of progressive politics; that values can provide a vital connection between the class interests central to eroding capitalism and other identity-interests with emancipatory aspirations; that the value of democracy should be accorded particular emphasis in relation to articulating a concrete programme of progressive politics; and that the overall plan of eroding capitalism is not state-centred. In the next chapter, Wright's more concrete agenda for accomplishing structural change will be addressed.

Sociologists can rarely predict events. In the paragraphs that follow my limited ambition is to draw from and apply aspects of the work of Abrams and Wright to propose what I see as the most likely social precursors to the structural change which I see, in turn, as a precondition for tackling health inequalities at home and abroad and for creating a *healthy society*. This idea of a healthy society is important. It denotes a society in which its citizens can – another of Bhaskar's favoured terms – 'flourish' individually and collectively.

Accomplishing transformative structural change in the UK

Given the current state of affairs in Britain, and for want of empirically credible alternatives, it seems probable that pressure sufficient to occasion structural change towards a better and more healthy society is most likely to arise in the form of Abrams' spontaneous mass mobilisation. In what follows I present what I see as an optimally viable scenario. I begin by once again stressing the role of the distinctive and potentially game-changing causal power of social class.

Class action: a necessary condition for structural change

The prevailing class structure in Britain and kindred countries diverges from that obtaining even a generation ago (see Box 4.2). Furthermore, class is multifaceted for all that it is its potent structural force that has been emphasised throughout this text. Class can and must be analysed as a lived experience as well as in terms of what Evans terms 'class on paper'. *Subjective* class, in other words, must be distinguished from *objective* class. Moreover, an inert class in-itself is far removed from an active and engaged class for-itself. To claim a high level of causal significance for class in relation to transformative structural change, therefore, requires considerable additional qualification and support. It will be argued here that class mobilisation remains a necessary – if not a sufficient – condition for the effectiveness of any spontaneous mass mobilisation; but for this necessary condition to be realised: (i) new cross-class alliances must be built, and (ii) this presupposes the overcoming of a plethora of hurdles induced not just by fragmentations in the class structure but by fractured society's pervasive cultural relativity.

Many sociologists are agreed on a growing fragmentation of the class structure, and for a number of neo-Marxists debates on how to define today's working class have become a preoccupation. It is apparent, however, that upward trends in post-2010 UK in underemployment and precarity, family and child poverty, homelessness, sickness and premature death have trespassed well into Evans' petty bourgeoisie and beyond into Wright's formerly stable middle class (that is, well into the 'squeezed middle'). The escalating cost of living crisis has breached today's more permeable class boundaries. It does not follow, of course, that this has or will translate into any kind of cross-class coalescence and the formation of a class-based social actor. Indeed, the imposingly high hurdle of cultural relativity might suggest otherwise.

The possibility of an emergent and expanded working class for-itself, however comprised, cannot yet be seen on the horizon. If it is right to claim that objective class has become more potent in rentier capitalism, undoubtedly subjective class has during this same period diminished its impact on identity-formation. While polls suggest people continue to be conscious of the class character of British society, this awareness has become 'lost' amid a fog of cultural 'clashes' and conflict that is functional for neoliberal ideology (in similar vein, Habermas maintained that postmodernism, qua cultural relativism, functioned to buttress the status quo, thereby constituting a form of neo-conservatism). As Wright recognises, people's sense of self or identity matters, but what has come to be called 'identitarian politics' has muddied the structural waters. It has led to a rapid inflation of individualised conflicts around who we are and might become, often linked to niche markets and increasingly fuelled by populist reactionary and right-wing political groups as a way of garnering support. Just as material cost of living quandaries have come to impact Evans' petty bourgeoisie and Wright's hitherto comfortable and stable middle class, so the politics of identity has transposed cultural quandaries onto and into the traditional working class. And the key point about cultural relativity is that it breeds scepticism and distrust about *all* rationally constructed narratives signalling and promoting the very idea of transformative social change.

On the face of it all this counts *against* regarding social class as a lever for transformative social change. And this prima facie pessimistic appraisal is reinforced by another observation. In his discussion of climate change, Huber (2022) makes the point that the most vigorous climate activists are overwhelmingly drawn from the university educated professional middle class (in the UK and Europe as well as in the US). So these activists are generally comfortable and secure inhabitants in high-income Western countries. Much the same might be said about activists protesting against war, contesting health inequalities and defending universal health care innovations like Obamacare and health systems like the NHS. With regard to climate change, Huber notes the tendency for these activists to furnish an agenda for 'de-growth' with a 'narrative of loss'. This, he sensibly writes, will clearly and unambiguously alienate *un*comfortable and *in*secure people struggling day-to-day to feed and clothe young children. It is a message, in other words, that is fundamentally incompatible with the pressing needs of many working-class families. Little wonder that there remains a propensity to neglect the message and shoot the messengers. The de-growth agenda for action on climate change is re-examined in Chapter Eleven.

My claim is that if emancipatory and transformative structural change is to occur in countries like Britain, then objective-to-subjective class action is a necessary condition, but that it now appears to be on the back foot. This understandable pessimism is countered in the subsections that follow.

Activity-convergence and a predisposition to anger and hatred

If there is a single emotion that leaks through permeable class boundaries in the UK it is likely to be public anger caused by the stress and distress of post-2010 political austerity and the descent into what seems at the time of writing to be an ever-deepening cost of living crisis. If this predisposition to indignation remains largely latent and contained within the private sphere of the lifeworld, this is doubtless a function of widespread anxiety and fatigue due to a protracted commitment to 'getting by'. The collapse of the UK's postwar 'social contract' has left millions of low-income families 'surviving not living'. Box 10.1 lists commonly expressed causes of anger in rentier capitalism.

Box 10.1: Common sources of public anger

- Significant and increasing wealth inequality, with no attempt to rein in the greed of the super-rich by a wealth tax or by tackling abuse through non-dom status or the use of tax havens.
- Openly encouraging super-rich and rich donors to buy policies from government that favour capital accumulation over meeting population needs.

- The discovery of 'magic money trees' to rescue private banks in 2008–09 while denying their existence when it comes to helping people struggling to get by.
- Executive abuse of parliament to circumvent scrutiny and accountability, with the passive connivance of parliamentary officials, including the Speaker of the House of Commons.
- Undemocratic musical chairs leading to a succession of 'unelected' Conservative prime ministers, culminating in Johnson's prevarications, the rapid implosion of Truss-economics, and the anointment of multimillionaire Sunak.
- The disastrous mishandling of the COVID pandemic, extending to the corrupt awarding of multiple contracts gifting public monies to unqualified private providers, often Conservative Party donors and friends.
- Continuing support for the full charity status of the leading 'public schools' and the Eton/Oxford route to high political office (chumocracy plus Oxocracy).
- Cutting back on welfare support via the introduction of Universal Credit.
- In the wake of a cost of living crisis exacerbated by Truss-economics, failing to control energy prices (the only country in Western Europe to do so), effectively allowing foreign-based private energy companies to enjoy new levels of profiteering reflected in obscene CEO salaries and dividends to shareholders.
- Looking the other way when private monopoly service providers exploit their customers (for example, transport).
- Favouring business cuts to labour forces, even at the cost of public safety, backed up by sanctions against people made unemployed if they do not pursue any part-time, zero hours 'bullshit jobs' in or outside the areas in which they live.
- Legislating to reduce trade union rights, despite incontrovertible evidence that strong trade unions are associated with more equal societies.
- Legislating to threaten and punish any citizens protesting against the removal of their rights or campaigning against unjust or oppressive government policies.
- The continued existence of a corrupt police force, readily available to repress the people on behalf of the government.
- The governmental privileging of profiteering over the futures of the people they purport to serve and the environment we and future generations share (for example, oil and fossil fuel production).

- Failing to build public or even affordable housing and condemning more and more people to substandard and hazardous accommodation and homelessness.
- Voting down Bills to ensure that all housing is 'fit for human habitation' and to put an end to 'no fault evictions' (more than 80 MPs rent out properties).
- Running down the NHS by means of a deliberate policy of underfunding to create sufficient public dissatisfaction with the health service to allow the government to send for for-profit providers (several Conservative and Labour MPs already have shares in private health care companies).
- The lack of any effective opposition from the Labour Party led by Starmer, who offer more of the same with a tweak or two.

In assorted combinations, there are plenty of items in Box 10.1 to excite very real public resentment and anger. And as Thomas Piketty (2014) has shown, such items, reflective of escalating inequality, represent capitalism 'working normally', not a passing and deviant phase. In fact, the era of the welfare state heralded by the election of Clement Attlee in 1945, and surviving up to the election of Thatcher in 1979, was the only 'passing and deviant phase' in living memory. The stigma/deviance dynamic is relevant here too. This is in part motivated by the class/command dynamic, whereby – as the result of a calculated political strategy – people who are poor and in dire straits are 'blamed for their shame': they are held to be personally and causally responsible for their circumstances. I have elsewhere referred to this as a 'weaponising of stigma' (Scambler, 2018a). If the charge of blame can be successfully appended to that of shame, then people are rendered 'abject' and are all the more prey to class exploitation and command or state domination. Some have internalised this charge of blame and their sense of 'felt stigma' and 'felt deviance' has blunted their anger. But this does not mean that their anger has altogether dissipated.

In his paper 'Toward a typology of mediated anger', Karin Wahl-Jorgensen (2018: 2071) argues that anger 'serves as a cause of engagement and a barometer of public feeling'. Identifying a spectrum, he contends that 'at one end sits rational and legitimate anger, which forms the basis for social change', while at the other is found illegitimate and irrational anger. Protesters can be simultaneously angry and rational, peaceful and legitimate. It is suggested here that widespread simmering public anger is both empirically affirmed and a significant and efficient fuel for, and input into, what has been called the 'protest sector of the public sphere' (Scambler and Kelleher, 2006). Anger, in short, falls into Abrams' categories of (psychological and) social affinities in relation to spontaneous mass mobilisation. In partial confirmation, a recent Norwegian study asked 2,000 adults how they felt about the climate crisis and found that the link to activism was seven times stronger for anger than it was for hope. When asked why they were angry, respondents most often said that it was because it was human actions that were causing climate change, especially those of politicians. Interestingly, however, fear and guilt emerged as the top predictors of policy support, while sadness, fear and hope were the best predictors of behavioural change (Gregersen et al, 2023).

In his critical examination of Marx and Engels' *Communist Manifesto*, initially published in 1848, China Mieville (2022) considers the current political role and potential of anger manifested as hate. That hatred can have a positive impact is not an easy case to make. But we inhabit a cruel rentier capitalist world, Mieville argues, that thrives on and encourages sadism, despair and disempowerment. Hatred on the part of the oppressed – among slaves, for example – is *inevitable*: it is far from productive to pathologise hate per se, not least when it arises naturally, let alone to make it a cause for shame. 'Class hatred' in the UK in the 21st century, this thesis runs, might be judged to have arisen naturally. This kind of hate is not a personal, psychological or pathological hate, 'but a radical structural hate for what the world has become'. Mieville (2022: 177) writes:

> The ruling class needs the working class. Its various fantasies of getting rid of them can only *be* fantasies, because as a class it has no power without those beneath it. Thus wider ruling-class contempt for the working class ('chavs'), thus class loathing, thus social sadism, thus the constant entitlement from the ruling class, that sense that they are special and that rules

don't apply, thus the deranged eulogising of cruelty and inequality. Vile as all this is, what it is not is *hate*, certainly not Aristotelian hate – because its object absolutely cannot be eradicated. For the working class, the situation is different. The eradication of the bourgeoisie *as a class* is the eradication of bourgeois rule, of capitalism, of exploitation, of the boot on the neck of humanity. This is why the working class doesn't need sadism, nor even revenge – and why it not only can, but must, hate. It must hate its class enemy, and capitalism itself.

So according to this 'update' of the manifesto of Marx and Engels, hate does indeed have a political function, that is, hatred of the system and its enduring structures, forces and tendencies. Class hatred is part of a complex set of arms and tools of resistance and can and must inform an effective strategy and push for transformative change. This is not, Mieville insists, to displace a rightful emphasis on love rather than hatred, *but it is to be realistic* ('realism 2' rather than 'realism 1', as cited earlier). It seems reasonable to summarise at this point by suggesting that hate might optimally: (i) be harnessed to motivate systemic and structural change, (ii) be used reflexively and strategically, and (iii) come second to love in any transition to a better, post-capitalist society. Love may be the natural currency of the lifeworld, but system rationalisation and colonisation brings with it a predisposition to anger and, ever lurking, a preparedness to hate.

A crisis of state legitimation

On the cusp of the switch to financialised or rentier capitalism, Jurgen Habermas (1975) published a somewhat neglected work entitled *Legitimation Crisis* (see Scambler, 2001). The analysis to this point has highlighted the likely significance of spontaneous mass mobilisation if transformative structural change in the UK is to be accomplished; nominated the working class as critical agents for guaranteeing the effectiveness of any such mobilisation, even while disabusing us of any notion that it presently exists as a class for-itself ready to act; and posited a neglected role for widespread public anger, and even hatred. The relevance at this point of Habermas' analysis is that a crisis of state legitimation seems the most probable way forces for change might be brought to a head.

Habermas' analysis of liberal capitalism is very largely Marxist, a perspective he later drifted away from and eventually abandoned. In the era of liberal capitalism, he argues in *Legitimation Crisis*, the logic, ethos and praxis of political economy seeped into, or more accurately 'stained', the everyday to-ing and fro-ing of interaction that constituted the fabric of the lifeworld. Capitalism provided not only for 'system integration' but for 'social integration'. Because of its contradictions, however, capitalism is always prone to economic crises. These can be frequent, following the natural course of the business cycle. In postwar liberal capitalism the state came to play an ever-increasing part in 'managing the economy' to offset these economic crisis tendencies. It monitored the likes of inflation and levels of employment, counteracting potentially damaging trends via policy shifts. It made welfare provision available, kept the heads of the unemployed above water, and slowed the downward spiral of overproduction by underwriting the unemployed as consumers. It also financed research and development. In short, it brought and maintained the unemployed 'inside' the system.

This enhanced role of the state, Habermas argues, represented a 'functional adaptation' within capitalism. It contained class conflict. But it also carried risks: with economic engagement came responsibility. Capitalism's crisis tendencies were not eliminated but rather displaced. The state picked up the tab. This opened up the possibility of what Habermas termed a 'rationality crisis', or a crisis that might be understood as emanating from the very philosophy of mediation adopted by the state. This philosophy promised to deliver economically while also retaining legitimacy re the electorate. It has been suggested that in the mid-to-late 1970s the state's Keynesian philosophy and approach came to be regarded as no longer 'fit for purpose', making a rationality crisis all the more likely.

A legitimation crisis occurs when the citizenry experiences a democratic shortfall, that is, when people feel under-represented. Habermas is aware that the 'formal' – parliamentary-style – democracy characteristic of modern highly differentiated societies falls well short of 'substantive' or participatory democracy. People know this and are generally content to let politicians go about their business. But people will on occasion rebel, notably when they come to regard those they elect too unaccountable to the electorate. So the state runs the risk of a rationality crisis if it fails to accommodate the demands of the economy, and a legitimation crisis if it fails to meet the demands of it citizens.

An additional type of crisis Habermas refers to as a 'motivation crisis'. This occurs when the culture of the lifeworld, in which what he calls civic privatism is embedded, falters. This transmutes into a risk when the social and cultural institutions of primary and secondary socialisation fail to produce and reproduce the work ethic. The 'imperative to work' is, of course, a basic premiss of capitalism, fuelling the subsystems of the economy (directly) and the state (indirectly). A weakening of the work ethic can render citizens, most especially young people, unresponsive or indifferent to this imperative.

This is a peculiarly perspicacious piece of theorising with clear ramifications for high-income countries such as the UK in rentier capitalism. Consider once more the breadth and depth of the UK's current crises. Dorling (2023: 21) summarises:

> The multiple crises that afflict Britain are worse and have deeper roots than those affecting other European states. The UK is now very likely to be the most economically unequal country in Europe (although until early 2022 it was ranked just slightly more equal than Bulgaria). The repercussions are widespread. It really matters that Britain has the most divisive education system in Europe, tainting our institutions and affecting individuals for life. It matters greatly that the UK has the most expensive and poorest-quality housing, the most precarious and often lowest-paying work for so many people, the lowest state pension and the stingiest welfare benefits. *Recently Britain has also experienced the sharpest declines in health in all of Europe, especially in the health of its children.* A whole state is being plunged ever deeper into poverty. This is failure [emphasis added].

He concludes that 'it is not surprising that even the rich are now worried'. In such circumstances it is not only unsurprising that anger and hatred can be cast among Abrams' affinities, but that an optimal route to structural challenge and change may well prove to be a crisis of state legitimacy. Rentier capitalism's neoliberal ideology has disarmed the state and undermined any Keynesian capacity to intervene. The state's survival through the 2008–09 financial crisis towards the close of Gordon Brown's New Labour regime was conceivably the last throw of its dice. Governmental austerity politics post-2010, culminating in the extraordinary self-detonating Truss-economics and its protracted aftermath, have brought the prospect of a legitimation crisis closer. Not only is there a ubiquitous public questioning of government competence and a leaking of confidence and trust, but there is a discernible lack of enthusiasm for Keir Starmer's purged Labour Party, which is not only providing weak parliamentary opposition but seems to have no alternative policy platform. Crises of rationality, legitimation and motivation may not be far off.

Trigger events

Spontaneous mass mobilisations draw on a series of affinities and convergences. The text of this chapter thus far has pointed to some of these that strike as especially pertinent in the UK in the 2020s. The next, I refer to as 'trigger events'. The thesis here is that it is likely to take a single unpredictable and isolated (that is, spontaneous) event to light the blue touch paper for the kind of impactful mass protest that is a precondition for deep and lasting change. These events can assume many different shapes and forms, so there is necessarily a limit to what can be said. In his discussion of the role of 'situations' in the structural conditions of convergence, Abrams (2023: 47) refers to 'paramount situations' when 'the structural obligation to participate can trump lingering fears or concerns people might have'. Such situations can be inspired by an array of factors, but Abrams stresses the importance of threat. He cites an incident in Egypt when mounted brigands charged into a peaceful protest in Tahrir Square, 'swinging swords at protesters and tossing Molotov cocktails into the crowds'. This repression immediately – spontaneously – backfired, with the result that 'scores of ordinary Egyptians poured forth into the streets to defend the revolutionary cause, remaining there for days to come'. As this case testifies, events that trigger spontaneous 'mass' mobilisations do not guarantee lasting structural change. Indeed, there are never guarantees. But for transformative social change to occur, the ducks of the causal prerequisites like those ventured here have to be in line.

Civil disobedience/violence

While few UK citizens would sign up to the view that all laws are warranted, there remains a deep-seated reluctance as well as trepidation at the prospect of flouting them. Moreover, what might be categorised as mild forms of activism, such as the 'slow walking' protests of the 'Just Stop Oil' protagonists, are now being heavily policed and overtly condemned by agents of an increasingly oppressive state. Marchers defending the NHS against privatisation, promoting rent controls, opposing continuing fossil fuel subsidies and 'Stop the War' activists calling for talks are, alike, being threatened with substantial fines and imprisonment. Holding up a placard has, in and of itself, been lambasted by statist defenders of the status quo. In other words, the state itself is trespassing beyond the 'symbolic violence' implicit in its defence of the status quo.

Bourdieu's notion of symbolic violence is important in this connection (see Burawoy, 2019). The state, he argues, is the site of a struggle to secure a monopoly of symbolic as well as physical violence. Symbolic violence is a form of what is often characterised as 'soft power'. The education system, for example, is a major conduit for the exercise of power over citizens. Arising out of his detailed empirical study of the French educational system, he concluded that it functioned to disguise the exercise of power and to reproduce existing power and class relations. It would be quite wrong to underestimate the potency of soft power. In my *Health and Social Change*, I posited the state-sanctioning and promotion of an adaptive, class-driven national 'habitus' or mindset in the UK from the 1970s, a mindset that gave succour to the new neoliberal ideology (Scambler, 2002). Currently, however, this longstanding political reliance on soft power is being complemented by a more coercive form of state power. The Public Order Bill builds on the public order measures in Part III of the Police, Crime, Sentencing and Courts Act of 2022. Among other things, it enables the police to impose conditions on a protest, provides for a statutory offence of intentionally or recklessly causing public nuisance, and increases the maximum penalty for the offence of wilful obstruction of a highway. It would be foolish to deny this well-documented drift towards a more authoritarian state, and sociologically naive to doubt that the police, and if necessary the armed forces, would be vigorously deployed in the event of a spontaneous mass mobilisation oriented to significant and lasting social change.

If the British state in rentier capitalism is acting first and foremost in the interests of monopoly capitalists, as is asserted in the class/command dynamic, while itself endeavouring to avoid a crisis of legitimation, and it is prepared to extend its soft or symbolic power to embrace more coercive types of policing, including violence, then this puts any discussion of the rights and wrongs of the civil disobedience and the violence committed by activists into context and perspective. Marx himself fleetingly hoped that the change he envisaged and campaigned for might be achieved in England by parliamentary means, but he was quickly disillusioned (Stedman Jones, 2017). In his *Parliamentary Socialism: A Study in the Politics of Labour*, Marxist Ralph Miliband (1991) also rejected the parliamentary route as unrealistic (and as the joke goes, had two sons to prove it). It is an analysis and point of view substantiated by the quick and decisive undermining of Jeremy Corbyn (and of Bernie Sanders in the US), and this despite the popularity of the measures contained in the Labour manifesto prior to the 2017 election. Evans (2023: 284) writes:

> Overwhelmingly, the Labour Party – and indeed, the labour movement – is represented in parliament and the media (and sometimes on the streets) by the professional-managerial classes – a strata of people who are (justifiably) the most widely detested people in society: people whose sense of their own superiority and self-righteousness is far more unacceptable to

working-class people than the traditional economic bourgeoisie or even the aristocracy.

Strong words with more than a germ of truth. The moral would seem to be not only that extra-parliamentary (spontaneous mass) mobilisations are critical, but that *working-class leadership* is paramount. This is another sub-theme that will be revisited later. Just as narratives of de-growth and loss will not galvanise the working-class re climate change, nor will professional/managerial class leadership re collective agency.

Utopian narratives

There is 'freedom from' and 'freedom to', and this distinction, as liberal philosopher Isaiah Berlin notably insisted in his inaugural lecture in 1958, embodies an important tension. My argument here is that spontaneous mass mobilisations sooner rather than later require a narrative addressing freedom *to* (achieve a richer, fairer and more caring lifeworld) as well as freedom *from* (the uncompromising travails of the class/command generated exploitation and bureaucratic domination of rentier capitalism). In practice this means: (i) distinguishing between 'utopian blueprints' that offer, to coin a phrase, oven-ready futures, and are almost invariably propagated by professional-class radical intellectuals and 'utopian realist' narratives that start from accessible critiques of the neoliberal status quo and are then constructed out of working-class grassroots activism; and (ii) 'scholarly texts' and 'manifestos', the former oriented to blueprint formats, and the latter to persuasions to engage and act.

In his Preface to the 1888 English edition of the *Communist Manifesto*, Engels wrote:

> When it was written we could not have called it a *socialist* manifesto. By Socialists, in 1847, were understood, on the one hand the adherents of the various Utopian systems: Owenites in England, Fourierists in France, both of them already reduced to the position of mere sects, and gradually dying out; on the other hand, the most multifarious social quacks

who, by all manner of tinkering, professed to redress, without any danger to capital or profit, all sorts of social grievances, in both cases men outside the working class movement, and looking rather to the 'educated' classes for support. Whatever portion of the working class had become convinced of the insufficiency of mere political revolutions, and had proclaimed the necessity of total social change, called itself Communist. It was a crude, rough-hewn, purely instinctive sort of communism; still, it touched the cardinal point and was powerful enough amongst the working class to produce the Utopian communism of Cabet in France, and of Weitling in Germany. Thus, in 1847, socialism was a middle-class movement, communism a working-class movement. Socialism was, on the Continent at least, 'respectable'; communism was the very opposite. And as our notion, from the very beginning, was that 'the emancipation of the workers must be the act of the working class itself', there could be no doubt as to which of the two names we must take. (quoted in Mieville, 2022: 244)

The concepts and emotions conjured up by the terms 'socialism' and 'communism' may be different in the 21st century, but Engels is making an important point that has a lively resonance here. Seeking to rehabilitate the idea of communism, the French philosopher Alain Badiou (2015) has advanced what he calls the 'communist hypothesis' in an attempt to reconceptualise the left. 'We know', he insists, 'that communism is the right hypothesis. All those who abandon this hypothesis immediately resign themselves to the market economy, to parliamentary democracy – the form of state suited to capitalism – and to the inevitable and 'natural' character of the most monstrous inequalities.' This was a universal call to arms.

Whatever the choice of words, there is a strong case for taking seriously the concept of communism advocated by Engels and Badiou. As Jamie Morgan (2022: 134) writes:

From our current geo-historical position, embedded in a growth system and socialised to think progress means a blanket commitment to more and more stuff in bigger and bigger economies (by exchange value), any radically different alternative seems alien and perhaps fantastical. But there is nothing natural about a capital accumulation system that puts profit before people and assumes human welfare can be an unintended consequence of a dynamic process of economic growth. This is just one form of social organisation, one that may appear uncoordinated but depends crucially on institutions that produce its possibility.

The idea of communism introduced here embodies a challenge not just to rentier capitalism's neoliberal ideology but also to Thatcher's iniquitous insistence that 'There Is No Alternative' (TINA).

It is incumbent on proponents of an alternative to rentier capitalism – whether under the rubric of communism or not – to disseminate a utopian realist narrative in manifesto form that: (i) eschews overly comprehensive blueprints, and (ii) is either (ideally) emergent from working-class leadership or (expediently) lends itself to working-class curiosity, adaptation and co-option. Insofar as the next chapter is an attempt to set out a few concrete ways to surmount the formidable obstacles to forging and inhabiting a 'healthy society', it might be said to offer a few tentative steps towards such a utopian realist narrative. The present chapter concludes with a warning. It has become commonplace to 'absent' considerations of the type epitomised by 'realism 2', that is, those considerations that 'realistically' confront the intimidating structural, cultural and agential obstacles to transformative change. There are many texts, for example, that establish sound principles of justice, democracy, 'sharing and caring' and so on with which action plans 'should' emerge. And there are others which lay out generalised policies which, if only they were enacted, would in and of themselves represent a fundamental shift in the social order (for example, the recommendations incorporated in the multiple national health reviews conducted by Marmot and others in the UK and globally by the WHO). It is not that critiques of the status quo or inputs solely at the level of philosophical principle or solely at the level of ideal(istic) policy recommendations are without value, far from it. It is rather that they end where we arguably should begin. As critical realists might put it, they 'absent' the more awkward issue of how significant social change might be accomplished *in the real world* and in the face of direct, and likely violent, resistance on the part of capital monopolists and their cross-class and state-recruited allies acting in accordance with the class/command dynamic.

ELEVEN

Policy, practice and obstacles

Every time a person in the Global South displaced by climate catastrophe or armed conflict migrates in search of shelter and a means of subsistence, every time someone in a high-income country such as the USA or the UK cannot access health care in an emergency, and every time foodbank users try to do so clandestinely for fear of the stigma weaponised against 'losers like them', then no sociological explanation for what is happening to them is complete without a micro-to-meso-to-macro-account of why they find themselves in such unnecessary and intolerable predicaments. We live in the UK in a fractured society, and one which is located in an increasingly fractured or shattered world. In his comprehensive review of the empirical literature, Danny Dorling (2023) refers to our 'shattered nation' and describes the UK as a 'failing state'. 'The UK', he writes,

> has been speeding in the wrong direction for over forty years and that has resulted in growing disillusion, despair and apathy. ... What may be helpful at this point is to realise that if there is no planned progressive change – change of the kind that last began in 1942 during the Second World War – then in each year from here on there will be more crises. (Dorling, 2023: 242–243)

Given the emphasis throughout this volume on the sheer causal power of prevailing social structures and cultural recipes in general, and of the ruling class or current hegemonic bloc in particular, this seems like a council of despair. But despair is not an option. This chapter visits general and specific policy options.

The ambitions of this contribution already extend well beyond typical considerations of sociology and health inequalities in fractured communities in the UK and across the globe. Having said that, they are nevertheless constrained, both by what it is possible to cover in a short volume like this and by my own limited expertise. I have addressed global inequalities of health and living and touched on climate change and the omnipresent threat of warfare in a rapidly changing world. I could have referred to so much more, such as the existence of a novel, up-and-running geopolitics of political and economic spying. Political scientists Henry Farrell and Abraham Newman (2023) have investigated what they call America's 'underground empire', a coercive US-led network allowing the US to eavesdrop on other countries, isolate its enemies and dominate trade (today's headlines about trade wars, sanctions and controls on technology exports are merely tremors hinting at far greater seismic shifts beneath the surface, as we sleepwalk into a dangerous new struggle for empire); artificial intelligence (AI), which is now being signalled as an imminent interruption to life as we know it; and the fact that we are likely to bequeath to future generations a 'post-human' existence (in his last, posthumous, work Stephen Hawking (2018) predicted that in a hundred years we will not recognise the human species as it now is). So climate change and war, global threats in their own right, are also used symbolically in this short pitch to make and illustrate the key point that examining the possibility of a healthy society raises issues at a structural and global level and well beyond those routinely addressed in standard sociologies of health inequalities.

If we are to reject TINA (There Is No Alternative), as we surely must, and not shirk from facing up to the very real obstacles to the displacement of predatory economic systems such as financial or rentier capitalism, then roadmaps to post-capitalist futures are required. In contemporary theoretical terminology, we must reassert power 1 relations and expeditiously disassemble those power 2 relations that stand in the way of individual and collective flourishing (Bhaskar); or commit ourselves to lifeworld decolonisation/rationalisation by stemming the insinuating and destructive flows of the subsystems' steering media of money and power that contaminate and poison everyday decision-making that is, in consequence, no longer anchored in communicative rationality (Habermas). An apt formula might draw on Wright's strategies. Wright was understandably wary of revolutions given the historical evidence of their past and always unpredictable sequelae, so an overall strategy might involve neutralising capitalism's harms as a calculated precursor to its structural transcendence and dismantlement.

I have referred elsewhere to a strategy of 'permanent reform', the underlying idea being that an escalating push to neutralise capitalism's harms might edge us a little closer to its structural transcendence, in the process bringing factors alluded to in Abrams' affinity-convergence model and in the overlapping theories and distinctions of Wright, Habermas and others into causal play (Scambler, 2018). I have also made a distinction between 'attainable' and 'aspirational' objectives of political engagement which is relevant here (Scambler, 2022a). It is a distinction that marries well with Wright's neutralising harms (attainable objectives) and structural transcendence (aspirational objectives); although even what were deemed attainable objectives a few decades ago now seem to be almost beyond reach. The kind of policy shifts on constitutional politics in the UK that I gave as examples included disabusing the monarchy of its obscene riches, tax privileges and clandestine political activity, on the grounds that 'trimming it' (with the aspirational objective of its ultimate abolition) would expose to critique a series of institutions that are parasitic upon it, such as hereditary aristocratic titles and entitlement, the House of Lords and a corrupted honours system that often functions as an extension of the Conservative Party. Further towards the aspirational end of the spectrum come the objectives of a new elected second chamber and full-blown republicanism.

In the economic domain I gave as examples of possibly attainable objectives the restoration of trade union rights, abolishing hire and rehire practices, ending zero hours contracts, increasing the minimum wage, increasing sick pay, replacing Universal Credit with a more supportive and less punitive benefits system, raising the UK's parsimonious state pension and restoring adequate funding to the NHS. Citing Christophers (2020), I mentioned reforming a taxation system which currently betrays an extreme 'rentier bent', for example through modifications to limit rentiers' ability to make excess profits and achievable via reducing the existing tax-based subventions supporting rentiers as well as increasing tax rates (and closing tax havens). More aspirational ambitions require more radical action. Piketty (2014) has estimated that the return on assets 'r' globally before tax has always been greater than the rate of economic growth 'g'; and for most of the history of capitalism, r after tax has also been greater than g, which leads him to claim that, *ceteris paribus*, wealth inequality increased under capitalism. Unusually after the Second World War, g exceeded net (post-tax) r, in the process curbing inequality, largely through a combination of 'exceptional growth' and progressive taxation policies. In rentier capitalism, Piketty argues for higher taxes on assets to bring r back below g to counteract surging wealth inequality. UK governments, Christophers (2020) adds, have 'featherbedded rentiers'. They have actively encouraged them via tax subsidies to be or become rentiers. Taxes on incomes earned from non-rentier activities could be lowered (utilising what economists call the 'negative reinforcement' dimension of taxation, namely, removing an aversive stimulus with the aim of strengthening what is judged a positive behaviour or outcome). Also, a tax on rentier assets and income streams could be introduced/increased (for example, a land-value tax).

In this chapter I take seriously the obstacles to the structural transcendence required for truly effective health-bestowing transformatory *and emancipatory* social change. Picking up on the research on education and social mobility conducted by Bukodi and Goldthorpe (2018) noted in the Introduction, the emphasis is firmly on equality of *condition* rather than equality of *opportunity*. I remain aware that there have always existed tensions inside and outside of Marxian frameworks around the phenomenon of the welfare state. On the one hand, as has been implicit through this contribution, stronger welfare states – like those found in Scandinavia – are associated with a reduced material and social inequality and a raised standard of living for the most disadvantaged. But on the other hand, precisely this move to level 'condition' functions to undermine opposition to capitalism as an economic and political system and mitigates against dissent and rebellion: capitalism is made to appear more palatable. Sartre makes a related point when he identifies a paradox. The French, he suggests, were never so free as when they were occupied by the Nazis in the Second World War. Bauman (2023: 169) summarises: we fall into enslavement through *the trap of coercion disguised as free choice*; but the occupiers made this trap inaccessible to the French who were left *without* a choice. These hard truths must perforce be borne in mind in any promotion and assessment of strategies oriented to transcending structures through permanent reform, neutralising harms and, just possibly, spontaneous mass mobilisation occasioned by a cost of living generated crisis of state legitimacy and a degree of structural rupture.

A note on the free flourishing of all

Many philosophers have attempted to provide both principles and warranties for creating the 'good society', most of them from within the liberal Western camp. This is not the place to review this extensive and often arcane literature, but it might be helpful to briefly sample Bhaskar's critical realist argument based on the concept of human flourishing. What Bhaskar refers to as the 'dialectic of freedom' is powered by the interface of absence and desire, since absence is a condition for desire (desire presupposes lack). Power 2 relations of the kind enshrined in the class/command and kindred dynamics stand in the way of the realisation of a complex array of human needs, as well as the pursuit of freedom (Sartre's trap of coercion disguised as free choice). Resisting and struggling against the sharper-edged forms of power 2 relations characteristic of rentier capitalism, and factoring in expanding cultural definitions of needs and wants constructed in part in the course of the struggle, 'nurtures and fuels a logic of more inclusive and encompassing definitions of and aspirations towards freedom' (Scambler, 2018a). This quotation from Bhaskar (1993: 263–264) is characteristic of his rather abstruse terminology, but it is worth including. It draws on his argument for 'absenting' those 'constraining ills' that power 2 relations embody:

Insofar as an ill is unwanted, unneeded and remedial, the spatio-temporal-causal-absenting or real transformative negation of the ill presupposes universalizability to absenting agency in all dialectically similar circumstances. This presupposes in turn the absenting of all similar constraints. And by the inexorable logic of dialectical universalizability, insofar as all constraints are similar in virtue of 'their being constraints', ie, qua constraints, this presupposes the absenting of all constraints as such. ... And this presupposes in its wake a society oriented to the free development and flourishing of each and all, and of each as a condition of all, that is to say, universal autonomy as flourishing. ... So the goal of universal human autonomy is implicit in every moral judgement.

In plainer language, in acknowledging and acting to negate the constraining ills that threaten our own concrete singularity, we are all as actors committed to acknowledging and acting to negate the constraining ills that threaten others who share common situations and a common human-social-being-in-nature (that is, concrete universalizability). The phrase 'common human-social-being-in-nature' has a special salience of course in the fields of national, regional and global health and health care, and in the context of the impending and potentially catastrophic threat of climate change and the scarcely more far-fetched nightmare of a possible thermonuclear conflict.

Overcoming obstacles to 'health and health care for all'

An agenda of permanent reform for accomplishing 'health and health care for all' which: (i) begins with neutralising the harms visited on us by financialised/rentier capitalism, and (ii) in which *(i) is a mere stepping stone to achieving the transformative and emancipatory structural change that is a precondition for the successful fulfilment of this agenda*, is no small task. It is important too to recognise that in campaigning for change we have no alternative but to start from where we are, and not from some more expedient but fantastical place. This agenda and task are vital both for health and health care in the UK and cross-nationally. First to be considered here is the health domain in England/UK.

The UK as a 'healthy society'

The early chapters of this book contained discussions of changes in population health and health inequalities in England/UK, and also addressed the policy recommendations advanced by a series of commissioned reports from the pioneering 'Black Report' – a model for its successors in that it fully costed its recommendations – to the more recent reports by Michael Marmot. In less detail, there was coverage also of changes in population health globally, culminating in policy changes commended by the World Health Organization (WHO). This kind of research and the type of policy set it bequeaths is certainly pertinent to neutralising harms. It is not unreasonable to suggest that it outlines plausible attainable objectives, while remaining obstinately abstract and nebulous around aspirational objectives: references to structural change are typically genuflecting add-ons. In what follows I offer some thoughts on key parameters for homing in on the kind of transformative structural change that I have argued is a precondition for improving population health, reducing inequalities and preparing the ground for more healthy societies.

A preliminary point is that we must escape the trap of coercion disguised as free choice by rejecting the conceptual framework that comprises a collective mindset functional for rentier capitalism's neoliberal ideology of TINA. There is a complex web of mythology to be debunked here. This involves contesting political/economic clichés such as appraising the individual economies of nation states via such putatively 'positive' indicators as accelerated growth and 'negative' indicators such as inflation and stagnation. This may seem counterintuitive, but such clichés lock us in to 'coerced' policy interpretation and decision-making that helps deliver structural continuity via the expediently false doctrine of TINA, a state of affairs that deflects public attention from the iniquitous consequences of the class/command and kindred dynamics. The 'growth versus de-growth debate' will feature later when climate change policy is considered. The necessarily schematic focus in this section will be on population health and health inequalities in the UK and on the nature of the NHS as a health care system.

There has been an upsurge of interest in and reflection on public health in general and on prevention in particular, both within the UK and internationally. In his recent piece in the *British Medical Journal*, Richard Smith (2023) repeats the familiar point that the NHS, like most health care systems, is oriented to disease not health; and he goes on to cite the WHO's definition of health as 'a state of complete physical, mental and social wellbeing and not merely the absence of disease or infirmity'. However, he is no fan of the WHO's definition, which he castigates as 'laughable, divisive, hierarchical and largely ignored'. What we need, he suggests, is to do away with the notion of prevention (that is, of disease) and to agree on a broader definition of health as 'something to do with resilience, adaptability, coping, interdependence, and relationships with others, our community, the planet, and nature'. We should forgo thoughts about health as being about individuals and recognise that it is 'something broader'. I should emphasise that Smith is not here using the notions of resilience, adaptability and coping as expressions of individual behaviour.

Making no claim for originality, I shall refer to the urgent need for a public health perspective that extends to challenging and transcending social and cultural structures (that is, one that focuses on aspirational objectives, or realism 2, in addition to attainable objectives, or realism 1). I shall refer to this as *a public health reformatted for constructing a healthy society*. A public health perspective and portfolio that restricts itself to – that is, stops at – attempting to neutralise harms is cutting off its nose to spite its face. A public health for making the UK a healthy society translates as increasing those flows of health-bestowing assets – namely, biological, psychological, social, cultural, spatial, symbolic and material assets – that are currently weakest and weakening in the working class and petty bourgeoisie. These, as argued earlier, constitute the prepotent media of enactment of class relations inside and outside the health domain. The causal chains involved are, of course, complex and have been extensively researched within the sociology of health and health inequalities (Bartley, 2016). But suffice to say that a known series of attainable-to-aspirational social interventions would undoubtedly combine to strengthen the asset flows of the working class (most conspicuously in the Midlands and the North of England) and Evans' petty bourgeoisie, relative, that is, to those of the more privileged classes. Examples of types of interventions building on those on worker and welfare rights and a re-oriented taxation system already mentioned might include the following, again on a spectrum from attainable to aspirational (see McDonnell, 2018). They do not add up to a policy programme for change, which is not possible here, but they do constitute an illustrative brief. The focus is on the promotion of equality: enough is known for us to be able to predict that *a more equal UK equates both with a healthier population and reduced health inequalities.*

- *Confronting inequality*: as has been documented here, the degree of wealth and income inequality in the UK has grown considerably since the 1980s. Furthermore, at the time of writing the Sunak government is actively considering scrapping inheritance tax, which is at present paid only by the top 3–4 per cent of wealth owners. Measures to curtail the greed of the 'greedy bastards' by rejigging taxes on wealth and income are not hard to fathom. For example: a tax on excess corporate profits; increased rentier taxation along the lines suggested by Christopers (mentioned earlier); a tax on financial transactions (for example, a Tobin-style tax); an increase in corporation tax (the UK rate is currently the lowest in high-income countries); the closing down of offshore tax havens; a phased increase in inheritance tax towards an aspirational target of 100 per cent; an increase in forms of progressive taxation (for example, the top rate of tax on earned income in the UK was 83 per cent in the 1970s, reduced to 60 per cent by Thatcher in 1980 and then to 40 per cent in 1989, increased to 50 per cent by Labour's Gordon Brown in 2010, and reduced once more by the Conservative/LibDem alliance to 45 per cent in 2013); and a decrease in regressive forms of taxation (for example, VAT). As far as welfare support is concerned, reversing the existing measure that halts financial support for families with more than two children tops many people's list as the optimal way of relieving child poverty. Increasing the state pension, abolishing Universal Credit and supplementing existing support for those most in need, especially those with disabilities, are paramount.

- *Promoting public housing*: shelter is a basic human need and one, in principle at least, easy to satisfy in a high-income country such as Britain. And yet, as Dorling (2023: 82–83) shows, 'housing precarity has been allowed to become so bad in the UK because it is in the interests of a small but very powerful minority of people'. What Dorling defines as 'the largest privatisation in British history' was the introduction of 'right to buy' by Thatcher. The 'unspoken aim' was to reduce the size of the social rented sector, which is why local councils were not permitted to use the money from the sale of council houses to build more council housing. What happened was that many of those who purchased their council houses at a big discount subsequently sold them on, often to private landlords who cashed in. Currently 87 MPs, 68 of them Conservatives, are landlords (that is, one in five Conservative MPs). Moreover, unacceptably poor housing conditions now extend beyond the private rental sector into not-for-profit housing associations. In the medium term we need to build more and better public housing stock, but in the interim, in a matter of months, we can reduce housing costs and precarity by making tenancy agreements more secure, by regulating rents, by taxing owners of multiple properties and by introducing more effective wealth taxes on housing than stamp duty.
- *Educating schools and universities*: Britain now has a fragmented amalgam of schools, mostly charged to communicate skill sets deemed appropriate to the perceived needs of the capitalist 'imperative to work'. In fact, a proper, worker-friendly introduction of robotics and AI can be plausible forerunners of a standard four-day working week backed by a universal basic income. The major public schools are insulated from the lower reaches of the job market. It is of critical importance that the grip of the public schools is loosened, and especially that the 'chumocracy' and 'Oxocracy' alluded to earlier are terminated. An obvious attainable objective would be ending the charitable status of the major public schools. It is critical for even the present stunted formal parliamentary democracy

that obtains in Britain that these institutions are brought into the state sector. All private schools need to be absorbed into a secular and comprehensive state system. The neoliberal business model deployed in universities must be abandoned, along with university fees and current pressures to restrict the funding of courses in the arts, humanities and social sciences. If not, then only the privileged Russell Group will be engaged in education – properly defined as 'intrinsically worthwhile' – as opposed to training. The Oxford/Cambridge axis, and the Oxocracy in particular, might be effectively disestablished by taking undergraduate teaching away from Oxbridge and making Oxford and Cambridge research institutions only.

- *Re-stabilising public utilities*: many Marxists have insisted that the logical endpoint of capitalism is the commodification of everything. If housing costs are most people's biggest expense, other 'unavoidable' costs include utilities like water, sewerage, phones, the Internet, fuel bills, transport and basic goods and services (for example, medicines). The fracturing of society in Britain has made accessing such items problematic. In the case of utilities this is largely a consequence of privatisation. A single private firm (Rothschild) was lead adviser or 'heavily involved' in the creation of 25 massive new private firms between 1988 and 1991 (British Steel in 1988, the ten UK Water Companies in 1989, the 12 electricity distribution boards in 1990, and British Coal and British Telecom in 1991). If this could be accomplished in so short a period, so too could its reversal. If an attainable objective is a stiffer regulation of privatised monopoly utilities, an aspirational one is their return to the public domain; this would cancel profiteering and drastically reduce prices. A free or low-cost 'integrated transport system' would cut car use, carbon dioxide (CO_2) emissions and other forms of pollution. Within the EU many of these options have already been taken.

- *Rescuing the NHS*: the NHS has been starved of funding post-2010 to rationalise its privatisation. Labour Party policy under Starmer differs little from that of the Conservatives. The point was made in the Introduction that health care systems contribute less to population health than is commonly assumed, but they retain a vital role. The NHS, especially in England, needs rescuing. The rhetorical cries for 'reform' typically reflect rentier capitalism's neoliberal ideology (as was the case over the privatisation of utilities). Insinuating for-profit providers into health care is regressive. If the NHS 'goes the American way', sacrificed on the altar of greed and money-making, we will look back fondly on the simple tripartite model enacted in 1948, for all its new-born imperfections. What the NHS requires is funding to address the current and growing gaps in provision, a commitment to general practitioners as efficient gatekeepers to expensive specialist care, above-inflation pay increases to retain its health workers, a paring down and rebooting of 'the new managerialism', and a long overdue re-commitment to its public health arm. Chronically overdue too is the creation of a National Social Care System to run alongside the NHS, as advocated in Jeremy Corbyn's Labour manifesto for the 2017 general election.

This quartet stands as an illustration of the kinds of attainable-to-aspirational objectives that are paramount for building a more equitable and fairer 'healthy society'. It is important to insist too that it is precisely such policies that are intrinsic to a 'public health reformatted for constructing a health society' and therefore fit for the 21st century. But how can these kinds of demands for UK change be squared with the preconditions for effective change globally?

Healthy societies in the 'periphery'

I have deliberately retained Wallerstein's term here because many low-income countries have been, and continue to be, dominated and exploited by the 'greedy bastards' in major transnational corporations anchored in, if not necessarily resident in or loyal to, core countries such as the US and UK. While the tectonic plates of the world-order might be shifting with the powerful emergence of China and India as major players, coupled with a few resurgencies within the semi-periphery, the lifeworlds of billions of citizens in peripheral countries remain obstinately defined by the hit-and-miss pursuit of those economic and social modes of subsistence left to them by system colonisation/power 2 relations. Moreover, these are pursuits made more hazardous by mass migrations now occasioned by climate change and warmongering. UNICEF and the Internal Displacement Monitoring Centre have reported that at least 43 million child displacements have been linked to extreme weather conditions over the last six years, with floods and storms accounting for 95 per cent of child displacements between 2016 and 2021 (Lakhani, 2023). The concept of asset flows posited here as pivotal for health and longevity in the UK can retain its salience in such circumstances in the periphery, *but it must be recontextualised.*

Where to begin in illustrating viable attainable-to-aspirational routes to the healthy society globally, with special applicability to the Global South? Acknowledging once more that we have no option but to start from where we find ourselves, we might begin with those global bodies that have emerged to ratify and consolidate capitalism through its various successive phases while continuing to facilitate its virile and predatory spread (see Box 1.1). Ian Golding (2013) recognises that contemporary processes of globalisation have 'left behind' many of those international institutions, such as the United Nations (UN), the International Monetary Fund (IMF) and the World Bank, that were intrinsic to capitalism in its previous incarnations. He writes that 'with new threats emerging from climate change, security crises, threats of global terrorism and cybercrime, pandemics, increased migration, and financial crises, global governance is crucial' (Golding, 2013: 173). The omens, he averred a decade ago, are not good. The UN, IMF and World Bank were 'overloaded' and no longer delivering; the 'small, informal directorate for managing the global economy that emerged in the 1970s', the G7, was outdated; and the other intergovernmental networks, like the G24 or G77 groups of developing countries, did not have the authority, the capacity or the legitimacy to deliver on 'the enormous expectations placed on them' (Golding, 2013: 173). He goes on to set out five principles for moving forward. The first: not all issues require global collective action. A principle of subsidiarity might apply, whereby some issues are resolvable at the national, regional or bilateral level, or by non-government actors. Second, he calls on a principle of selective inclusion, whereby only key actors are engaged, namely, countries with the most power to effect solutions and countries most affected by the problem. Third comes a principle of variable geometry, dictating that only a minimum of countries required at each stage of managing a problem are engaged: different countries engaging on different issues, and at different stages of global action. The fourth principle is one of legitimacy: any rules of engagement must be understandable and acceptable to most countries. And finally, there must be some degree of enforceability at the global level: governments must do as they promise.

Golding's principles are helpful but, like most other discourses in this field, they betray an awareness of the dynamics of class and power *without facing up to their consequences*. How to surmount the ubiquitous profiteering of nomadic capital monopolists who hold national governments to ransom? How to undo the use of national and international aid packages that function to procure cheap labour for transnational corporations, to impose private finance initiatives, or simply to export Western-style consumerism to sell stuff, even health-damaging products banned in high-income countries? How to stop leading pharmaceutical companies who use pandemics like COVID to exploit publicly funded university research to maximise the return on their vaccine patents, quite independently of need? An Oxfam report entitled 'Prescriptions for Poverty' described drug companies as 'tax dodgers, price gougers and influence peddlers'. Their research found that four pharmaceutical companies – Abbott, Johnson & Johnson, Merck & Co and Pfizer – 'systematically stash their profits in overseas tax havens', and that they 'appear to deprive developing countries of more than $100 million every year – money that is urgently needed to meet the health needs of the people in these countries – while vastly overcharging for their products'. These activities 'exacerbate the yawning gap between rich and poor, between men and women, and between advanced economies and developing ones' (Oxfam, 2018: 4–5). It often seems that commentators are more comfortable espousing liberal principles than in staring the likes of the class/command dynamic and its global penetration in the face. It is not as if journalists in the mainstream media in countries such as Britain are much bothered.

Walden Bello (2002: 107) perspicaciously borrows from Thomas Kuhn's (1962) *Structure of Scientific Revolutions* to note that when a paradigm is in crisis – in the present context, neoliberal economics – there are one of two responses. He writes:

> One is that followed by the adherents of the old Ptolemaic paradigm, which was to make more and more complicated adjustments to their system of explanation until it became too complex and virtually useless in promoting scientific advance. The other path was that taken by the partisans of the new Copernican system, which was to break away completely from the old paradigm and work within the parameters of the competing paradigm, which could not only accommodate dissonant data in a far more simple fashion but also point to new exciting problems.

To reiterate a constant theme, the myth of TINA has to be debunked. As Bello rightly goes on to acknowledge, however, this is no easy task. New systems cannot be constructed without weakening the hold of the old. As argued in the previous chapter, he too emphasises the importance of a legitimation crisis. But what is also required is a strategy embracing a 'deconstruction' of the old system *and* a 'reconstruction' of the new. Without regurgitating the theories of the previous chapter, Bello's schemata fits in well with them.

In terms of deconstructing 'oldthink', Bello (2002) insists that any strategy must respond to 'the needs of the moment'. He was writing over 20 years ago, but he then insisted that the 'anti-corporate globalisation movement' must limit the brief and powers of the World Trade Organization, expressly to halt trade liberalisation. Activists should work with national movements, such as peasant movements for food sovereignty in the Global South and citizens' movements in the Global North, to press their governments to stop further liberalisation in agriculture, services and other areas. Ultimately, what was required was a 'global critical mass' with real momentum. 'Newthink', representing processes of reconstruction, would for Bello prefigure a new form of global governance epitomised by his idea of a double movement of deglobalisation, focusing on both: (i) national economies, and (ii) a pluralist system of global economic governance. While the idea of deglobalisation derived mostly from the experience of societies in the South, it is relevant also to the Global North. At its core is a strategy for reorientating economies away from an emphasis on production for export to production for the local market. In more detail this would mean:

- drawing most of a country's financial resources for development from within rather than becoming dependent on foreign investment and foreign financial markets;
- implementing long postponed measures of income and land redistribution to forge a vibrant internal market that would become the anchor of the economy and create the financial resources for investment;
- de-emphasising growth and maximising equity in order to radically reduce environmental disequilibrium;
- not leaving strategic economic decision-making to the market but making them subject to democratic deliberation and choice;
- subjecting the private sector and the state to constant monitoring by civil society;
- creating a new production and exchange complex that includes community cooperatives, private enterprises and state enterprises, and excludes transnational companies;
- enshrining the principle of subsidiarity in economic life by encouraging production of goods to take place at the community and national level if it can be done at a reasonable cost in order to preserve community (adapted from Bello, 2002: 113–114).

It is an approach that consciously subordinates the logic of the market, the pursuit of cost efficiency, to the values of security, equity and social solidarity: it is about re-embedding the economy in society rather than having society driven by the economy. In other words, it espouses lifeworld rationalisation and decolonisation (Habermas) and the reassertion of lifeworld-oriented power 1 over those system-oriented power 2 relations that issue in 'constraining ills' (Bhaskar). But Bello was under no illusions about the formidable nature of the obstacles to achieving such a social structural transformation: 'The reigning god ... is a jealous one that will not take lightly challenges to its hegemony' (Bello 2002: 114).

In fact, this kind of transformation is only possible if it takes place within an alternative global economic governance. This necessarily means greatly reducing the power of the Western-based transnational corporations that are the main drivers of globalisation and the political and military hegemony of the states, most conspicuously the USA, that protect them. What is required is not an alternate set of centralised global institutions, but instead a deconcentration and decentralisation of institutional power and the creation of 'a pluralistic system of institutions and organisations interacting with each other, guided by broad and flexible agreements and understandings' (that is, not unlike the period from 1950 to1970 under the auspices of the General Agreement on Tariffs and Trade).

Climate change and the healthy society

In many respects the climate crisis has overtaken orthodox thinking about health inequalities at home and abroad. It is a crisis that must sit at the heart of any credible public health paradigm and programme fit for purpose. But it has at the same time refocused attention on the most compelling causal powers implicated in this 'new' and dire planetary threat; and these powers overlap significantly with those underpinning UK and global material and social inequalities. Mark Maslin (2021) rightly observes that a quartet of inter-related challenges need addressing simultaneously: climate change; environmental degradation; global inequality and extreme poverty; and global, national and individual security. We have the technology and the resources, he argues, but we need to: update our international institutions; redesign economics for real people; develop a new geopolitics for the 21st century; set meaningful global targets; and develop pathways to our shared future. The omens, to reiterate, are discouraging. As far as climate change is concerned, we have seen that coal is the largest contributor to CO_2 emissions. The US is the fourth largest producer of coal worldwide (595 million tonnes in 2022), but despite the fact that 45 big global insurers have adopted policies limiting coal underwriting in recent years, a report by the campaign group Insure our Future found that loopholes are being exploited and companies are violating their own policies. In fact, Lloyds of London is the second biggest underwriter of US coal (Kollewe, 2023).

In their discussion of the urgent necessity of moving from 'personal responsibility' to an 'eco-socialist state', Erin Flanagan and Dennis Raphael (2022) argue that despite the evidence that social democratic states such as Denmark, Finland, Norway and Sweden have responded proactively to climate change through environmental policies that complement public policies promoting economic and social security, even these eco-socialist welfare state environmental policies are unlikely to avert a climate catastrophe. What is required, they contend, is: 'gaining public control over energy policy and countering the power and influence of fossil-extracting industries. In theory, this could be accomplished through existing policy instruments. In reality, it may require establishment of a post-capitalist eco-socialist state, the outlines of which remain uncertain even among leading eco-socialist scholars' (Flanagan and Raphael, 2022: 244). The authors go on the define an eco-socialist state as a system run by institutions of the state which prevent concentrations of power among private interests like fossil fuel giants, and instead provides an expansion of democracy to the public so that the working class is able to govern themselves (in stark contrast, they add, to the socialism of the Soviet and current Chinese eras). Eco-socialism, then, involves democratic ecological planning and the suppression of economic actors operating in their own interests who are unapologetically polluting the environment. These two Canadian academics advocate nationalising fossil fuel and related industries and placing them in the service of controlling climate change. It is an argument that sits comfortably with a growing advocacy of a form of 'green socialism' that involves a shift not only away from fossil fuel capitalism but away from capitalism itself by bringing under public control energy, water and other utilities, expanding public sector services, adopting principles of economic democracy and socialising investment (Carroll, 2021). They cite George Monbiot (2022) approvingly: 'Only a demand for system change, directly confronting the power driving us to planetary destruction, has the potential to generate effective action.'

This is to affirm what might be characterised as the recurring and central 'double-thesis' of this book, namely: (i) that a radical socio-structural transformation is a precondition for effectively addressing UK and global health inequalities, climate change and the constantly evolving threat of warfare, and (ii) that it is precisely the present structural configuration that is intimidating and stopping sociologists and others from facing up to this. This is an issue to be directly dissected in the next and concluding chapter.

A pivotal concept under discussion by those assessing options to deal with climate change, which is now superimposed on the challenge of dealing with global, regional and national health inequalities, is that of *de-growth*. Reference was made earlier to the recovery of some of Marx's late and unpublished writings touching on this. Saito (2023: 23) writes:

> The richness of nature in the form of land, water, and forests is obviously indispensable for human flourishing as means of subsistence and production as well as for a healthy life. ... 'The Earth is the reservoir, from whose bowels the use-values are to be torn'. This statement is consistent with Marx's recognition of the essential contribution of nature to the production process: 'Labour is not the source of all wealth. Nature is just as much the source of use values (and it is surely of such that material wealth consists'!) as labour.

Nature, it might be said, enters the labour process and aids in the production of commodities alongside workers, but without entering the valorisation process as it is not a product of labour. Nature is free and capital sets out to utilise its power as much as possible. Use value is subordinated to exchange value under the capitalist logic of valorisation. The result is the destruction and squandering of nature and what was earlier defined as metabolic rift.

Saito comments on the opposition of abundance and scarcity. Regardless of how much capitalism increases the productive forces, this opposition – this 'paradox of wealth' – does not disappear but is instead intensified due to the constant creation of artificial scarcity. *It is not necessary to maximise productive forces to overcome this kind of scarcity.* 'Marx's de-growth communism aims to repair the "irreparable" metabolic rift and to rehabilitate the non-consumerist "abundance" of the social and natural wealth' (Saito, 2023: 226). De-growth communism promises to produce less both to lessen the burden on the natural environment and also to increase free time. Saito (2023: 235) again:

> When Marx argued that humans can organise their metabolic interaction with the environment in a conscious manner, it means that they can consciously reflect upon their social needs and limit them if necessary. This act of self-limitation contributes to a conscious downscaling of the current 'realm of necessity' which is actually full of *unnecessary* things and activities from the perspective of well-being and sustainability. They are only 'necessary' for capital accumulation and economic growth and not for the 'all-round development of the individual'. Since capital drives us towards endless consumption, especially in the face of 'the *total absence* of identifiable *self-lim*iting targets of productive pursuit admissible from the standpoint of capital's mode of social metabolic reproduction' (Mészáros, 2012: 257; emphasis in the original), self-limitation has a truly revolutionary potential.

Kate Soper (2023: 183) likewise insists that we need to 'dissociate pleasure and fulfilment from intensive consumption, from the endless accumulation of new machines and gadgetry'. She advocates an 'alternative hedonism' and concludes that we must rethink the good life. We need, Saito exhorts: (i) to shift from profit to use-values; (ii) to reduce the working day; (iii) to transform the remaining realm of necessity to increase workers' autonomy and make work more attractive; (iv) to substitute de-growth communism and a deacceleration of the economy for the market competition for profits; and (v) to overcome the antithesis between mental and physical labour. According to Saito, Marx regarded these five transformations as prerequisites for achieving a post-capitalism social formation.

In similar vein, Klaus Dorre (2018: 246) argues that we need a global debate 'on the contours of a democratic, egalitarian, non-capitalist, post-growth society'. He lays out four essential projects. The first involves 'scientifically' attacking systemic mechanisms which promote permanent destructive growth, which implies a rupture with superfluous consumerism. Second, we need substantive equality because ecological sustainability cannot be achieved without social sustainability. This means a radical redistribution from the North to the South, 'from top to bottom, from the strongest to the weakest' ('the 60 million refugees of whom only a small fraction actually reach the capitalist centres, for example'). Third, no redistribution will occur without a 'radical rebellious democracy' to take on 'the 1,318 companies currently controlling four fifths of the global economy'. And finally, Dorre makes the compelling point that each of these three can only succeed on a global scale, and this demands global cooperation in relation to ecological threats, economic crises, refugee movements and wars.

It has been maintained throughout this book that the social structural and cultural obstacles to accomplishing aims and objectives like these are deeply obstructive and well defended. Class warfare has often transmuted into the prosecution of armed inter- and intranational interventions. I have pointed to possible resistance and change in the form of the emergence of conditions favourable to spontaneous mass mobilisations. It remains only to recall and reinforce Huber's (2022) compelling argument discussed earlier, namely, that: (i) a structural transformation will not be accomplished by protests and dissent on the part of the professional classes – and that includes the authors cited here, and me – but must be rooted in and emerge from a collective working-class praxis, and (ii) the very idea of a post- or de-growth communist economy *will not mobilise the working classes if it is premised on 'a narrative of loss'* (they have insultingly little in a rabidly unequal world to be asked to make sacrifices).

Warfare and the healthy society

Humans have never been strangers to violence, even among the hunter-gatherers, though what is currently understood as warfare is a more recent phenomenon. And wars and the insecurities they visit on populations and the individuals that comprise them remain a constant into the 21st century. When I started drafting this text the Russians were in the process of invading Ukraine, and now as I near its completion Hamas has just launched a brutal attack on citizens in Israel, and Israel has responded with the sustained bombing of Palestinian infrastructure and citizenry in Gaza that is already being classed as a 'war crime'. In a moment of profound irony, Putin is charging the Western powers with the sanctioning of mass and inhuman violence on the part of Netanyahu's regime. The preceding chapters have expounded on the linkages between material and social equality and sustainability and their salience for a healthy society.

Dyer (2021) rehearses the by now familiar refrain that any remedial action or measures must start from where we are and not where we would like to be. Amid the plethora of current threats, he contends, the international system is undergoing a process of adjustment to the rise of new great powers and the relative decline of most of the existing powers. 'The ticket to superpower status in the world of 2040 will be brutally simple: only countries of subcontinental scale with populations near to or over half a billion people.' Specifically, the US, China and India. We have no option other than solving the problem of war within the multilateral system we have been building since the Second World War. The UN Charter gave the five victorious powers – the US, the UK, France, the Soviet Union and China – permanent seats on the Security Council, while other countries have to rotate through on two-year terms. To sanction military action against a country accused of aggression, the quintet of core powers must convince enough temporary members to gain a majority vote in the 15-member Security Council. But any one of the core powers can veto action, even if the majority in favour is fourteen-to-one. As of March 2022, Russia/USSR had used the veto 120 times, the US 82 times, the UK 29 times, France 16 times and China 16 times. Trials for war crimes were also introduced after the Second World War. They have a chequered history. The relative failure of the institutions of the UN is in part because it comprises poachers turned gamekeepers. Wrongly I think, Dyer blames the failures of the UN and other international bodies less on national governments than on the people they – nominally – serve. What he sees as people's 'enormous domestic resistance to any surrender of independence', I would interpret in terms of system colonisation and ideological obfuscation (which in rentier capitalism has taken a neoliberal form).

The UN Charter's ban on changing borders by force has had some successes and some notable failures. Failures include the eight-year war between Iraq and Iran in the 1980s (deliberately prolonged by American and Russian aid to Saddam Hussein in the hope that he would topple the revolutionary Islamic regime in Iran), and the illegal Soviet invasion of Afghanistan in 1979 and the US-led invasion of Iraq in 2003. The UN has no mandate to intervene in the multiple civil wars, many of them in Africa. Nor is the UN proving effective in the ongoing armed conflict between a relentlessly colonising Israeli state and Palestinian rights. While there are no ready-made solutions to ongoing armed conflict, what seems incontrovertible is that severely reducing global inequality, committing to the ubiquitous combatting of climate change and underwriting more sustainable ways of constructing the good, or healthy, society make credible and effective action more probable.

This chapter has necessarily offered a truncated discussion of a series of major geopolitical quandaries. If solutions have been hard to come by, it has revealed that these cannot be solved within the system which is rentier capitalism. System rationalisation or colonisation in the UK as elsewhere continue to hold multiple lifeworlds in its thrall. In particular, the capitalist monopolists, or greedy bastards, who steer the biggest of the transnational corporations are proven enemies of constructive policies and practices. Witness their self-serving and destructive behaviours in the boardrooms of the fossil fuel industry, arms sellers and in Big Pharma for example. But there will be those in and around the sociology community in the UK and further afield that judge the implicit agenda of this and the preceding chapters to be overly ambitious, ill-advised, misdirected or simply unacceptable.

TWELVE

The future: whither sociology?

A healthy society according to the precepts of this volume is one in which there no longer exist extremes of material and social inequality; greater equality is not achieved domestically at the price of dominating, exploiting and exporting inequality to semi-peripheral and peripheral societies; there is urgent, appropriately phased action against climate change, but not involving loss for the poorest and most disadvantaged nationally, regionally and globally; and in which the society makes a discernible and effective effort to enhance individual security at home and abroad by pursuing peace. Britain is manifestly not a healthy society by these criteria, and less so in post-1970s rentier than in postwar welfare state capitalism. There are some signs that public health thinking is changing, however. For example, Dina Von Heimburg and colleagues (2022) commend reconceptualising the field of public health as a public good. They advocate universal wellbeing as an organising principle for the economy. This sees economic systems as mechanisms to serve the common good and safeguard public interests rather than pursuing growth 'as a mission in its own terms':

> A wellbeing economy values and monitors what really matters for people to matter and flourish. This recognises that investing in social sustainability and 'leaving no one behind' is vital for achieving the wider aspects of sustainable development. Wellbeing economy is therefore about making investments in public goods such as health, education, nature and

vibrant communities, where local neighbourhoods represent the basic unit of sharing, caring and democratic empowerment. (Von Heimburg et al, 2022: 1064)

They go on to specify the need for comprehensive programmes of global action, local action and people action:

These three interdependent areas of action are vital to co-create a persistent drive pushing forward required and transformative social change: a comprehensive societal movement for the common good, where key public values are safeguarded and promoted through a system-wide approach to human rights and the SDGs [the UN's Sustainable Development Goals]. (Von Heimburg et al, 2022: 1068)

But what remains missing from these admirable aspirational objectives (realism 1) is any sense of the intricate economic and geopolitical potency of the obstacles to their realisation (realism 2). And this is where sociology might/should contribute to the debate.

There will undoubtedly be sociologists of health, illness, wellbeing and health care systems who instinctively disagree with the arguments advanced in this book, so this concluding chapter focuses on the rightful role of the sociologist. Let me be clear what my standpoint amounts to. Consider once more Burawoy's (2005) four basic types of sociology outlined in Box 1.3, namely, scholars committed to *professional* sociology, reformers delivering on *policy* sociology, radicals offering *critical* sociology, and democrats venturing into *public* sociology. *I affirm the importance of each of this quartet,* and especially professional sociological scholarship, which forms the basis of all we can offer the wider community via descriptive, explanatory and deliberative incursions into Habermas' public sphere of the lifeworld. I am here very much indebted to the studies and analyses of professional, policy, critical and public sociologists of health inequalities, whom I am nevertheless about to criticise! And my criticism is rooted in Bhaskar's notion of 'absence', or what they neglect to confront, or even avoid confronting.

In a paper published in 1996, I drew on the work of Habermas to set out a rationale for doing sociology (Scambler, 1996). I articulated this by means of five theses. First, I argued that sociologists had yet to come to terms with the enhanced or hyper-reflexivity of what I called 'high' modernity (I then and now felt/ feel uncomfortable with the more predictive 'late' modernity). Sociologists, in other words, were slower grasping life in a society characterised by accelerating change – Archer's 'morphogenetic society' – than they often appreciated.

Second, sociologists needed to be more aware and reflexive about its primary allegiances to economy and state and, via the steering media of money and power, to system rationalisation/ colonisation. I argued that sociologists had grown more responsive to short-term system needs than to the far-reaching effects of changes in UK welfare and health policy for the lifeworld. Much research, for example, was then (and is now) devoted to service audit and evaluation. My point was not that such projects were intrinsically undesirable, but rather that their engineered and disproportionate pursuit had to be understood in the context of an impetus to economic privatism and statist authoritarianism. Sociologists had 'adjusted themselves to' newly optimal flows of largely commissioned research funding. The result was 'a pattern of enquiry and research consonant with, or at least not *effectively* opposed to, the imperatives of economy and state' (Scambler, 1996: 575).

The third thesis insisted that sociology's principal commitment is to the rationalisation of the lifeworld, a commitment that is, of course, inconsistent with a primary allegiance to system needs. The system ties of sociologists of health and health care, I maintained, not only functioned to constrain their research options but led them to communicate almost exclusively to system-based or 'established intellectuals', rendering them either witting agents of manipulation in the lifeworld or unwitting agents of systematically distorted communication; either way, I wrote, 'their work serves strategic action and lifeworld colonisation rather than communicative action and lifeworld rationalisation' (Scambler, 1996: 575).

Following on from this, the fourth thesis was that sociology's principal commitment to lifeworld rationalisation required its promotion of and engagement with a *reconstituted* public sphere of the lifeworld. Britain was characterised then as now by a 'formal' parliamentary democracy, or in the phrasing of Habermas (1975: 36), by 'a legitimation process that elicits generalised motives – that is, diffuse mass loyalty – but avoids participation'. Since social and health policy priorities are framed by private investment decisions in the subsystem of the economy, politics is democratic in form only; thus, it is largely irrelevant which political party holds office since the state's commitment endures – administering the economy so that crises are avoided. Formal democracy can be contrasted with 'substantive' democracy, which allows for the genuine participation of citizens in the process of will-formation. Substantive democracy serves to institutionalise in the public sphere the *fundamental* norms of rational speech and discussion. Substantive democracy, Habermas claimed, entails further rationalisation of the lifeworld via the reconstitution of the public sphere out of the residue of a 'bourgeois public sphere' that was once progressive and resistant to economy and state, but which had collapsed into 'a sham world of image creation and opinion management in which the diffusion of media products is in the service of vested interests' (Thompson, 1995: 177). Fated to be actors in high modernity, I suggested, sociologists must, if they are to realise a predominant commitment to lifeworld rationalisation, *necessarily* engage with a reconstituted public sphere. Burawoy's commendation of 'public sociology', represented by those I call 'democrats', is pertinent here. Democrats must seek answers to the following question

> of whether, and to what extent, a public sphere dominated by mass media provides a realistic chance for the members of civil society, in their competition with the political and economic invaders' media power, to bring about changes in the spectrum of values, topics, and reasons channelled by external influences, to open it up in an innovative way, and to screen it critically. (Habermas, 1992: 455)

It is an issue that Habermas (2023) has revisited in light of the introduction of the Internet and of social media.

My final thesis was that if sociology is to be effective in promoting and engaging with a reconstituted public sphere, it must build alliances with (arguably) system-based and (especially) lifeworld-based activists.

The five theses elaborated in this paper, written a quarter of a century ago, stand as a prolegomenon to the arguments of this volume and, I would suggest, retain traction. Recalling Bhaskar's concept of 'absence', they highlight what sociology was and is *not* doing as opposed to what it was and is doing. It is in this context that I extended Burawoy's four types of sociology by appending a further duo: *foresight sociology* practised by *visionaries* and oriented to alternate futures, and *action sociology* practised by *activists* and oriented to making change happen. These are sociologies and sociologists who have always existed but on the margins of the discipline. Defending and emphasising the importance of their roles and contributions is pivotal to this whole text (see also Scambler, 2018). Consider once more the fact/value distinction. It was earlier argued that sociology's descriptive and explanatory incursions into the social world cannot be so easily circumscribed by this distinction as has often been assumed. Values seep into many studies, as if by osmosis. Sociologists of health and health inequalities in Britain, for example, typically assume that if medical interventions are proven effective (for example, hip and knee replacements), they *should* be made available to the whole population, and if health inequalities can be defined as inequities, then action *should* be taken to reduce or eliminate them. The gap between the high-income Global North and the low-income South *should* be addressed, as *should* the worldwide risk of climate change and the continuing propensity for armed conflict. Moreover, it is almost a given that opposition to these 'shoulds' *should* be exposed and circumvented or combatted.

Ruth Levitas (2013) in her *Utopia as Method* shows how far contemporary sociology has travelled from its classical beginnings. Much of classical sociology was geared to securing the good society, for all that it often remained caught up in an 'unreconstructed' European Enlightenment project marked by a radically classed and gendered colonialism: it was bourgeois, masculine and white. What Habermas (1984, 1987) argues for is a 'reconstructed' – de-classed, de-gendered and de-racialised – version of this 'project of modernity' (Scambler, 1996, 2001). Picking up on Levitas' discussion, what is sociology about *and for* if it demands neutrality in the face of rentier capitalism's predatory capital monopolists and its deepening intra- and international exploitation and disharmony, now hovering on the edge of dystopia and with the threat of worse to come via a collapse in planetary wellbeing? This is *not*, to repeat myself, to undermine any of professional, policy, critical and public sociologies, nor is it to require that all sociologists switch allegiance to foresight or action sociology. But it is to argue that members of the international sociological community should cover the bases of all six types of sociology. We should *between us* devote more attention to an evidence-based foresight sociology of optimal or superior alternative organisations, institutions and modes of governance and an evidence-based action sociology of exposing, resisting and overcoming capital- and power-based opposition. The neophyte sociology of climate change is now beginning to encourage more excursions into foresight and action sociology than hitherto, the sociology of health and health inequalities less so to date.

The neo-liberalisation of universities in the UK and elsewhere is often proving antithetical to the development of impactful foresight and action sociologies, including in the fields of health, health inequalities and health care. I have considered why and how this is so in a discussion paper with two colleagues (Scambler et al, forthcoming). We highlight the manner in which universities are being compelled by system imperatives to compete; staff are facing both individual competition and growing job precarity; old wheels are constantly being reinvented as individuals are harried into ever higher rates of productivity; specialisation – for example, theory and research as silo-like discrete areas and discourses – is easing out cross-fertilisations and interdisciplinarity; bureaucratisation via a metrics of accomplishment is privileging fund-raising for increasingly commissioned research projects over theoretical innovation; cultural relativity, the onset of cancel culture and identity politics are undermining longstanding philosophies of science and social science; and practitioners like sociologists are experiencing an enhanced degree of anomie or normlessness. In other words, the omens, as so often in the current era, are less than auspicious, and it has grown harder than it was for the babyboomer generation of sociologists to respond positively to the foresight and action sociology agendas commended here. Paradoxically, it has got harder as the need has grown more compelling.

Muckraking sociology in the health field

A case might be made across all six types of sociology that what studies in the health field lack is the input of *muckraking sociology*. It will not have escaped the attention of readers of this volume that much of the latest and more telling data were supplied by investigative journalists rather than sociologists or other academics. This is in part a function of speed of entry to the lifeworld's public sphere via today's innovative platforms. But it also comprises a challenge to sociologists to: (i) make greater use of these platforms (and to be recognised and rewarded institutionally for doing so), and (ii) to 'get their hands dirty' by committing to what Gary Marx (1972), in more receptive times, called 'muckraking sociology'. He cites from the first issue of *Transaction* in 1963: 'the social scientist studying contemporary problems and the complex relationships among modern men knows that he can no longer discharge his responsibilities *by retreating from the world until more is known*' (Marx, 1972: 1; emphasis added). Setting to one side the outdated sexist language, it remains relevant to ask if sociology in the UK, and indeed elsewhere, is in retreat on matters of overriding public salience and concern, such as those providing the foci for this book. Muckraking sociology, according to Marx (1972: 2), 'documents conditions that clash with basic values, fixes responsibility for them and is capable of generating moral outrage'.

The term muckraking derives from 'muckrake', an instrument used for gathering dung into a heap. In the hands of investigative journalists, muckraking came to be identified with uncovering and exposing misconduct on the part of prominent individuals and the collation of incriminating evidence. A lengthy quotation from Marx (1972: 3) is warranted here:

> Such research uses the tools of social science to document unintended (or officially unacknowledged) consequences of social action, inequality, poverty, racism, exploitation, opportunism, neglect, denial of

dignity, hypocrisy, inconsistency, manipulation, wasted resources and the displacement of an organisation's stated goals in favour of self-perpetuation. It may show how, and the extent to which, a dominant or more powerful class, race, group or stratum takes advantage of, misuses, mistreats or ignores a subordinate group, often in the face of an ideology that claims it does exactly the opposite. In pointing out a state of affairs that strikingly clashes with cherished values, muckraking research may have an expose, sacred cow-smashing, anti-establishment, counter-intuitive, even subversive quality, for it grows out of and helps sustain social upheaval and questioning. Although sociology like any other intellectual undertaking always has this potential, it is often not realised.

Could Marx's explication of muckraking have any more bite than it does here? The sheer enduring obstinacy of intra- and international material, social and health inequality, the out-of-control momentum of climate change and the rampaging suffering caused by worldwide armed conflicts – at the time of writing epitomised in the Gaza massacres – surely demand exposing and holding to account those who surf abiding social structures and facilitative cultures to their personal advantage and the disadvantage of millions, even billions, of generally anonymous others.

It was commonplace in the 1960s to ask of fellow sociologists, 'Whose side are you on?'. Marx suggests that sociology's involvement with public issues might in fact be cyclical. For American sociologists, he points out, the 1960s signalled the unfortunate involvement in Southeast Asia, and in part consequence there developed a reciprocal relationship between critical social science and social movements. Cyclical or not, there is a strong case that the time is ripe to extend the sociological project to expose and critique ideological obfuscation. Moreover, it is tempting to speculate that the ongoing conflict between an Israel backed by the US and its allies and, nominally, Hamas, but in reality a captive Palestinian population in Israeli-occupied Gaza (in which Hamas is embedded) – which at the time of writing has graduated to the sustained Israeli bombing of Gaza resulting in mass civilian deaths – might invite a re-asking of the question, 'Whose side are you on?'. What is incontrovertible is that practitioners of muckraking sociology are needed to examine the whys and wherefores of the complex regional geopolitics involved, and which companies based in which countries are selling sophisticated weapons systems to which buyers for use by whom in which countries. Enough is known already for us to hypothesise that the profits of the capital monopolists and their allies and shareholders rank higher than even child death tolls in the thousands.

Social structures and relations like those of class and command that causally deliver institutions that exploit and oppress, it is contended here, are not just legitimate phenomena to be studied and theorised by sociologists, but *should* also be called out and opposed, possibly in alliances not just with 'established intellectuals' (that is, via insiders and realism 1) but also with 'movement intellectuals' (that is, via outsiders and realism 2). While sociologies of people's health and health care systems provide a lens through which to view society and social order and change, the reverse is no less true. There currently exists a deficit not only in the macro-level or 'big sociology' of health phenomena, but, even more starkly, in what Levitas (2013) conceptualises as 'utopia as method' and its foresight and action concomitants.

Final thoughts

In this contribution to an important and continuing area of sociological interest and engagement, namely, social dimensions of health and health care, the idea of a 'healthy society' has afforded a critical subtext. In a series of publications dating back a quarter of a century I have upbraided colleagues in sociology as well as public health for merely mentioning and not confronting and taking on the causal power of those social structures most relevant for social pathologies in distributions of population health and systems of healing. Often their reluctance to do so can be traced to one or more of institutional intimidation; relatedly, individual reputational or career security or advancement; and an understandable desire to improve things via piecemeal social engineering. I can appreciate all this, but I hope here to have introduced and illustrated some strong reservations. In his *The Existential Moment*, Patrick Baert (2017) draws on the philosophy and actions of Sartre during the Second World War as a way of developing a general account of 'intellectual collaborationists'. Sartre himself argued that collaboration is ubiquitous, a normal phenomenon to be found across all societies. It is rooted, he thought, in social disintegration. Baert (2017: 86) writes:

> For Sartre, the collaborator conflates what is with what ought to be by submitting himself to the 'reality' of the present. He promotes an 'ethics of virility', attributing a moral dimension to the contemporary constellation simply by virtue that it managed to force itself upon us. The collaborator embraces a fallacious 'historicism' in which history is portrayed as a tale of progress, with the present as a necessary improvement on the past. He projects himself into the future and claims that, from the point of a distant future, the then-present state of affairs – with its collaboration – would make perfect sense and would be justified because by then the criteria by which we judge political events and decisions will be substantially different. Armed with this perverse logic of historicism and 'realism', the collaborator evades the responsibilities of the present. By looking at the present from the perspective of a distant future, the present is portrayed as the (future) past and stripped of its intolerable features. Once portrayed as a past, the present becomes abstract and no longer something to be lived through.

On the face of it, it seems more than far-fetched to draw parallels between a France occupied through the Second World War and any kind of appraisal of health sociology. And indeed, even the most neoliberal and demanding of the UK's universities do not equate to the Nazi occupation of France! But there are lessons to be learned. There are routes to collaborationism many of us have been exhorted to tread within (and even beyond) Burawoy's quartet of types of sociologies of health and health care. In a blog

I ventured a handful of ideal types of sociological collaborationism (see www.grahamscambler.com/blogs). The first was 'careerism', involving, beyond very understandable strategies for survival, *the sacrifice of integrity* in pursuit of personal advancement. Careerism best epitomises collaborationism and poses the greatest risk to the sociological project. The second was 'normalisation', indicating a wilful attempt to 'pass' or to 'cover' – heads below the parapet – *but this in neoliberal times*. The third was termed 'avoidance', exposing a wilful but contrived tactic of skirting around or avoiding the debunking of myths and the challenging of ideologies that *should*, indeed *must*, be the very bread and butter of sociological practice. This often involves choosing to engage only with 'uncontroversial' issues. I went on to contrast the *bystanders* who fail to challenge the status quo with the *subversives* who are willing to face down rentier capitalism's plutocrats. These are challenges we sociologists in the health domain face *as a community*.

References

Abrams, B. (2023) *The Rise of the Masses: Spontaneous Mobilisation and Contentious Politics*. Chicago: Chicago University Press.

Ahmed, N. (2022) Rishi Sunak's family profiting from ties to oil giant Shell. *Byline Times*, 19 July.

Ahmed, R., Atun, R., Burgand, G., Castro-Sánchez, E., Charani, E., Ferlie, E. B. et al (2021) Macro level influences on strategic responses to the COVID-19 pandemic – an international survey and tool for national assessments. *Journal of Global Health* 1 July.

Arbuthnott, G. and Calvert, J. (2021) *Failures of State: The Inside Story of Britain's Battle with Coronavirus*. London: Harper-Collins.

Archer, M. (2007) *Making Our Way in the World*. Cambridge: Cambridge University Press.

Austin, J. (1962) *How to Do Things with Words*. Oxford: Oxford University Press.

Badiou, A. (2015) *The Communist Hypothesis*. London: Verso Books.

Badiou, A. and Engelmann, P. (2019) *For a Politics of the Common Good*. Cambridge: Polity Books.

Baert, P. (2017) *The Existentialist Moment: The Rise of Sartre as a Public Intellectual*. Cambridge: Polity Press.

Bambra, C., Lynch, J. and Smith, K. (2021) *The Unequal Pandemic: Covid-19 and Health Inequalities*. Bristol: Policy Press.

Barrett, J. (2023) As Thames Water sinks, Macquarie Group continues its unstoppable rise. *Guardian*, 10 July.

Bartley, M. (2016) *Health Inequality: An Introduction to Concepts, Theories and Methods* (2nd edn). Cambridge: Polity Press.

Bauman, Z. (2007) *Liquid Times: Living in an Age of Uncertainty*. Cambridge: Polity Press.

Bauman, Z. (2023) *My Life in Fragments*. Cambridge: Polity Press.

Beck, U. (1982) *Risk Society*. London: Sage.

Beck, U. (1999) *World Risk Society*. Cambridge: Polity Press.

Bello, W. (2002) *Deglobalisation: Ideas for a New World Economy*. London: Zed Books.

Bhaskar, R. (1975) *Realist Theory of Science*. Hassocks: Harvester Press.

Bhaskar, R. (1987) *The Possibility of Naturalism: A Philosophical Critique of the Human Sciences* (2nd edn). Hemel Hempstead: Harvester Wheatsheaf.

Bhaskar, R. (1989) *Reclaiming Reality: A Critical Introduction to Contemporary Philosophy*. London: Verso.

Bhaskar, R. (1993) *Dialectics: Pulse of Freedom*. London: Verso.

Black, D., Morris, J. and Townsend, P. (1982) Inequalities in Health: The Black Report. In Townsend, P. and Davidson, N. (eds): *The Black Report and the Health Divide*. Harmondsworth: Penguin.

Blakeley, G. (2023) Time to make the climate profiteers pay. *Tribune*, 1 August.

Borras, A. (2020) Towards an intersectional approach to health justice. *International Journal of Health Services* 51: 206–225.

Brewer, M. (2019) *Inequality: What Do We Know and What Should We Do About It?* London: Sage.

Bright, S. (2023) *Bullingdon Club Britain: The Ransacking of a Nation*. London: Byline Books.

British Medical Association (2022) Health funding data analysis. Available from: www.bma.org.uk/advice-and-support/nhs-delivery-and-workforce/funding/health-funding-data-analysis

British Medical Association (2022a) NHS hospital beds data analysis. Available from: www.bma.org.uk/advice-and-supp ort/nhs-delivery-and-workforce/pressures/nhs-hospital-beds-data-analysis

British Medical Association (2022b) NHS backlog data analysis. Available from: www.bma.org.uk/advice-and-support/nhs-delivery-and-workforce/pressures/nhs-backlog-data-analysis

Brown, G. and Harris, T. (1978) *Origins of Depression*. London: Tavistock.

Bukodi, E. and Goldthorpe, J. (2018) *Social Mobility and Education in Britain*. Cambridge: Cambridge University Press.

Burawoy, M. (2005) For public sociology. *American Sociological Review* 70: 4–28.

Burawoy, M. (2019) *Symbolic Violence: Conversations with Bourdieu*. Durham, NC: Duke University Press.

Byrne, D. and Ruane, S. (2017) *Paying for the Welfare State in the 21st Century*. Bristol: Policy Press.

Campbell, D. (2021) Private hospitals treated just eight Covid patients a day during pandemic. *Guardian*, 7 October.

Carrington, D. (2023) Humanity at the climate crossroads: highway to hell or a liveable future? *Guardian*, 20 March.

Carroll, W. (2021) Conclusion: Prospects for Energy Democracy in the Face of Passive Revolution. In Carroll, W. (ed): *Regime of Obstruction: How Corporate Power Blocks Energy Democracy*. Vancouver: UBC Press.

Centre for Health and the Public Interest (2021) For Whose Benefit? NHS England's Contract with the Private Hospital Sector in the First Year of the Pandemic. London: CHPI.

Christophers, B. (2020) *Rentier Capitalism: Who Owns the Economy, and Who Pays for It?* London: Verso.

Christophers, B. (2023) *Our Lives in Their Portfolios: Why Asset Managers Own the World*. London: Verso Books.

Christophers, B. (2023a) Our new financial masters: how asset managers work in the shadows – and shape all our lives. *New Statesman*. Available from: www.newstatesman.com/ideas/2023/04/our-new-financial-masters

Chun-Han, L., Nguyen, L., Drew, D., Warner, E., Joshi, A., Graham, M. et al (2021) Race, ethnicity, community-level socio-economic factors, and risk of COVID-19 in the United States and the United Kingdom. *Lancet* 38 (https://doi.org/10.1016/j.eclinm.2021.101029).

Coburn, D. (2000) Income inequality, social cohesion and the health status of populations: the role of neo-liberalism. *Social Science and Medicine* 58: 41–56.

Coburn, D. (2009) Inequality and Health. In Panitch, L. and Leys, C. (eds): *Morbid Symptoms: Health Under Capitalism*. Pontypool: Merlin Press.

Commonwealth Fund (2023) US health care from a global perspective, 2022: accelerating spending, worsening outcomes. Issue Briefs, 31 January.

Cook, R. (2017) The firm with a back door key to Number 10. *The Independent*, 7 April.

Creaven, S. (2007) *Emergentist Marxism: Dialectical Philosophy and Social Theory*. London: Routledge.

Declassified UK (2023) The UK's 83 Military Interventions Around the World Since 1945. London: Declassified UK.

Dodd, V. (2023) Black people were three times more likely to receive Covid fines in England and Wales. *Guardian*, 31 May.

Dorling, D. (2023) *Shattered Nation: Inequality and the Geography of a Failing State*. London: Verso.

Dorre, K. (2018) *Growth, Degrowth or Post-Growth? Towards a Synthetic Understanding of the Growth Debate*. Berlin: Forum New Economy.

Doyal, L. and Doyal, L. (1999) The British National Health Service: a tarnished moral vision. *Health Care Analysis* 7: 263–276.

Drever, F., Doran, T. and Whitehead, M. (2004) Exploring the relation between class, gender and self-rated general health using the new socioeconomic classification: a study using data from the 2001 census. *Journal of Epidemiology and Community Health* 58: 590–596.

Dyer, G. (2021) *The Shortest History of War*. Exeter: Old Street Publishing.

El-Gingihy, Y. (2018) The great PFI heist: the real story of how Britain's economy has been left high and dry by a doomed economic philosophy. *Independent*, 16 February.

Elias, N. (1969) *The Civilising Process: The History of Manners and State Formation and Civilisation*. Oxford: Blackwell.

Elkins, C. (2005) *Imperial Reckoning*. New York: Henry Holt.

Elkins, C. (2022) *Legacy of Violence: A History of the British Empire*. Oxford: Bodley Head.

Evans, D. (2023) *A Nation of Shopkeepers: The Unstoppable Rise of the Petty Bourgeoisie*. London: Repeater Books.

Farrell, H. and Newman, A. (2023) *Underground Empire: How America Weaponised the World Economy*. London: Allen Lane.

Fitzpatrick, R. and Chandola, T. (2000) Health. In Halsey, A. and Webb, J. (eds): *Twentieth Century British Social Trends*. London: Macmillan.

Flanagan, E. and Raphael, D. (2022) From personal responsibility to an eco-socialist state: political economy, popular discourse and the climate crisis. *Human Geography* 16: 244–259.

Fooks, G., Mills, T., Mullan, K., Yates, D. and Willmott, J. (2023) How Britain's Covid support for big business entrenched inequality. *openDemocracy*, 30 May.

Foster, J. (2000) *Marx's Ecology: Materialism and Nature*. New York: Monthly Review Press.

Fraser, N. (2019) *The Old Is Dying and the New Cannot Be Born*. London: Verso Books.

Galbraith, J. (1992) *The Culture of Contentment*. London: Sinclair-Stevenson.

Garrett, P. (2019) What are we talking about when we talk about 'Neoliberalism'? *European Journal of Social Work* 22: 188–200.

Garton-Crosby, A. (2023) The Tory donors with links to fossil fuel interests and climate denial. *The National*, 31 July.

Golding, I. (2013) *Divided Nations: Why Global Governance Is Failing and What We Can Do About It*. Oxford: Oxford University Press.

Goto, R., Guerrero, A., Speranza, M., Fung, D., Campbell, P. and Skkauskas, N. (2022) War is a public health emergency. *Lancet* 399: 1302.

Gough, I. (2017) *Heat, Greed and Human Need: Climate Change, Capitalism and Sustainable Wellbeing*. Cheltenham: Edward Elgar.

Graeber, D. and Wengrow, D. (2021) *The Dawn of Everything: A New History of Humanity*. Oxford: Blackwell.

Greener, I. (2022) The 'New Five Giants': conceptualising the challenges facing societal progress in the twenty-first century. *Social Policy and Administration* 56(1).

Gregersen, T., Andersen, G. and Tvinnereim, E. (2023) The strength and content of climate anger. *Global Environmental Change* 82 (https://doi.org/10.1016/j.gloenvcha.2023.102738).

Grover, C. (2019) Violent proletarianization: social murder, the reserve army of labour and social security 'austerity' in Britain. *Critical Social Policy* 39: 335–355.

Gurr, T. (1970) *Why Men Rebel*. Princeton, NJ: Princeton University Press.

Habermas, J. (1975) *Legitimation Crisis*. London: Heinemann.

Habermas, J. (1984) *Theory of Communicative Action, Volume 1: Reason and the Rationalisation of Society*. London: Heinemann.

Habermas, J. (1987) *Theory of Communicative Action, Volume 2: Lifeworld and System: A Critique of Functionalist Reason*. Cambridge: Polity Press.

Habermas, J. (1992) Further reflections on the public sphere. In Calhoun, C. (ed): *Habermas and the Public Sphere*. Cambridge, MA: MIT Press.

Habermas, J. (2023) *A New Structural Transformation of the Public Sphere and Deliberative Politics*. Cambridge: Polity Press.

Harvey, F. (2023) Phase down of fossil fuel inevitable and essential, says Cop28 president. *Guardian*, 13 July.

Hawking, S. (2018) *Brief Answers to the Big Questions*. London: Bantam Books.

Hood, C., Gennusco, K., Swain, G. and Catlin, B. (2016) County health rankings: relationships between determinant factors and health outcomes. *American Journal of Preventive Medicine* 50: 129–135.

Horton, H. (2023) Fossil fuels received £20 billion more UK support than renewables since 2015. *Guardian*, 9 March.

Horton, R. (2020) *The Covid-19 Catastrophe: What's Gone Wrong and How to Stop it Happening Again*. Cambridge: Polity Press.

Horton, R. (2020a) Richard Horton: 'It's the biggest science policy failure in a generation.' *Financial Times*, 24 April.

Huber, M. (2022) *Climate Change as Class War*. London: Verso.

Hyde, M. and Rosie, A. (2012) World systems theory and the epidemiological transition. In Scambler, G. (ed): *Contemporary Theorists for Medical Sociology*. London: Routledge.

Ingleby, F., Woods, L., Atherton, I., Baker, M., Elliss-Brookes, L. and Belot, A. (2021) Describing socio–economic variation in life expectancy according to an individual's education, occupation and wage in England and Wales: an analysis of the ONS Longitudinal Study. *Social Science and Medicine – Population Health* 14: 100815.

International Energy Agency (2022) Global Energy Review: CO_2 Emissions in 2021. IEA.

Jolly, J. (2021) Serco brazens out Covid calamity as the profits roll in. *Guardian*, 18 April.

Joseph Rowntree Foundation (2023) UK Poverty 2023. London: JRF.

Khilnani, S. (2022) The British Empire was much worse than you realise. *The New Yorker*, 28 March.

King's Fund (2021) Key Facts and Figures about Adult Social Care. London: King's Fund.

King's Fund (2022) What are health inequalities? Available from: www.kingsfund.org.uk/publications/what-are-health-inequalities

King's Fund (2022a) The NHS budget and how it has changed. Available from: www.kingsfund.org.uk/projects/nhs-in-a-nutshell/nhs-budget

Kleinman, A. (1985) Indigenous Systems of Healing: Questions for Professional, Popular and Folk Culture. In Salmon, J. (ed): *Alternate Medicines: Popular and Policy Perspectives*. London: Tavistock.

Kollewe, J. (2023) Big European insurers 'underwrote 30% of US coal despite net zero pledges'. *Guardian*, 28 September.

Kuhn, T. (1962) *Structure of Scientific Revolutions*. Chicago, IL: Chicago University Press.

Kuper, S. (2022) *Chums: How a Tiny Caste of Oxford Tories Took Over the UK*. London: Profile Books.

Lakhani, N. (2023) Extreme weather displaced 43m children in past six years, Unicef reports. *Guardian*, 6 October.

Launchbury, C. (2021) Grenfell, race, remembrance. *Wasafiri* 36: 4–13.

Launer, J. (2023) Talking Point: a generation betrayed. *BMJ* 381: 901 (https://doi.org/10.1136/bmj.p901).

Levitas, R. (2013) *Utopia as Method: The Imaginary Reconstitution of Society*. London: Palgrave Macmillan.

Lewis, S. and Maslin, M. (2015) Defining the Anthropocene. *Nature* 519: 171–180.

Leys, D. and Player, S. (2011) *The Plot Against the NHS*. London: The Merlin Press.

Lofland, J. (1978) *The Craft of Dying: The Modern Face of Death*. Beverley Hills, CA: Sage.

Lyotard, J.-J. (1984) *The Postmodern Condition*. Manchester: Manchester University Press.

Marmot, M. (2006) *Status Syndrome*. London: Bloomsbury.

Marmot, M., Allen, J., Goldblatt, P., Boyce, T., McNeish, D., Grady, M. et al (2010) Fair Society, Healthy Lives: Strategic Review of Health Inequalities in England Post-2010 (The Marmot Review). London: Department of Health.

Marmot, M., Allen, J., Goldblatt, P., Herd, E. and Morrison, J. (2020) Build Back Fairer: The COVID-19 Marmot Review. The Pandemic, Socioeconomic and Health Inequalities in England. London: Institute of Health Equity.

Marx, G. (ed) (1972) *Muckraking Sociology: Research and Social Criticism*. London: Routledge.

Maslin, M. (2021) *How to Save Our Planet: The Facts*. London: Penguin.

Maugham, J. (2023) *Bringing Down Goliath*. London: W. H. Allen.

Mays, N. (2018) Health Care Systems. In Scambler, G. (ed): *Sociology as Applied to Health and Medicine*. London: Palgrave.

McCartney, G., Bartley, M., Dundas, R., Vittal Katikireddi, S., Mitchel, R., Popham, F. et al (2019) Theorising social class and its application to the study of health inequalities. *Social Science and Medicine – Population Health 7*.

McDonnell, J. (ed) (2018) *Economics for the Many*. London: Verso.

McGuire, B. (2023) I thought the government's plan to protect Britain from extreme heat would be bad. It's worse than that. *Guardian*, 20 July.

Medvedyuk, S., Govender, P. and Raphael, D. (2021) The reemergence of Engels' concept of social murder in response to growing social and health inequalities. *Social Science and Medicine* 289: 114377.

Mészáros, I. (2012) *The Work of Sartre: Search for Freedom and the Challenge of History*. New York: Monthly Review Press.

Mieville, C. (2022) *A Spectre Haunting: On* The Communist Manifesto. London: Head of Zeus Ltd.

Milanovic, B. (2015) Global inequality of opportunity – how much of our income is determined by where we live? *The Review of Economics and Statistics* 97: 452–460.

Miliband, R. (1972) *Parliamentary Socialism: A Study in the Politics of Labour*. London: Merlin Press.

Monbiot, G. (2020) The government's secretive Covid contracts are heaping misery on Britain. *Guardian*, 21 October.

Monbiot, G. (2022) Days of rage. Available from: www.monbiot.com/2022/07/19/days-of-rage

Morgan, J. (2022) Andrew Sayer on Inequality, Climate Emergency and the Ecological Breakdown: Can We Afford the Rich? In Sanghera, B. and Calder, G. (eds): *Ethics, Economy and Social Science: Dialogues with Andrew Sayer*. London: Routledge.

Mortimer, I. (2014) *Centuries of Change*. London: Bodley Head.

Murphy, R. (2023) Sunak is turning up the heat and the anger may be hard to constrain. Funding the Future Blog, 1 August.

Niranjan, A. (2023) 'Era of global boiling has arrived', says UN chief as July set to be the hottest month on record. *Guardian*, 27 July.

NOAA National Centres for Environmental Information (2023) State of the Climate: Global Climate Report for 2022. Available from: www.ncei.noaa.gov/access/monitoring/monthly-report/global/202300

Office of National Statistics (ONS) (2022) Trend in life expectancy by National Statistics Socio-economic Classification, England and Wales: 1982 to 1986 and 2012 to 2016. London: ONS.

Oldenburg, R. (1989) *The Great Good Place*. Boston, MA: Da Capo Press.

Omran, A. (1971) The epidemiological transition: a theory of the epidemiology of population change. *Millbank Memorial Quarterly* XLIX: 509–538.

openDemocracy (2023) Revealed: taskforce to tackle NHS backlog is stuffed with private health CEOs. London: openDemocracy.

Oxfam (2018) Prescriptions for Poverty. London: Oxfam.

Piketty, T. (2014) *Capital in the Twenty-First Century*. Boston, MA: Harvard University Press.

Platt, L. (2021) Covid-19 and ethnic inequalities in England. *LSE Public Policy Review* 1: Article 4.

Pollock, A. (2005) *NHS Plc: The Privatisation of Our Health Care*. London: Verso.

Rex, J. (1973) *Race, Colonialism and the City*. London: Taylor & Francis.

Riley, C. (2023) *Imperial Island: A History of Empire in Modern Britain*. London: Penguin Random House.

Riley, M. (2020) Health inequality and COVID-19: the culmination of two centuries of social murder. *British Journal of General Practice* 70: 397.

Ritzer, G. (2003) *Contemporary Sociological Theory and its Classical Roots*. New York: McGraw-Hill.

Roderick, P. and Pollock, A. (2022) Dismantling the National Health Service in England. *International Journal of Social Determinants of Health and Health Services* 52: 470–479.

Roser, M. (2021) Global economic inequality: what matters most for your living conditions is not who you are, but where you are. London: Our World in Data.

Sagan, C. (1983) Global atmospheric consequences of nuclear war. *Science* 222, March.

Saito, K. (2017) *Capital, Nature and the Unfinished Critique of Political Economy*. New York: Monthly Review Press.

Saito, K. (2023) *Marx in the Anthropocene*. Cambridge: Cambridge University Press.

Savage, M. (2015) *Social Class in the 21st Century*. London: Pelican.

Sayer, A. (2005) *The Moral Significance of Class*. Cambridge: Cambridge University Press.

Sayer, A. (2015) *Why We Can't Afford the Rich*. Bristol: Policy Press.

Scambler, G. (1987) Habermas and the Power of Medical Expertise. In Scambler, G. (ed): *Sociological Theory and Medical Sociology*. London: Tavistock.

Scambler, G. (1996) The 'project of modernity' and the parameters for a critical sociology: an argument with illustrations from medical sociology. *Sociology* 30: 567–581.

Scambler, G. (ed) (2001) *Habermas, Critical Theory and Health*. London: Routledge.

Scambler, G. (2002) *Health and Social Change*. Buckingham: Open University Press.

Scambler, G. (2018) *Sociology, Health and the Fractured Society: A Critical Realist Account*. London: Routledge.

Scambler, G. (2018a) Heaping blame on shame: 'weaponising stigma' for neoliberal times. *Sociological Review* 66: 766–782.

Scambler, G. (2019) The Labour Party, Health and the National Health Service. In Scott, D. (ed): *Manifestos, Policies and Practices: An Equalities Agenda*. London: UCL Press.

Scambler, G. (2020) *A Sociology of Shame and Blame: Insiders Versus Outsiders*. London: Palgrave.

Scambler, G. (2020a) COVID-19 as a 'breaching experiment': exposing the fractured society. *Health Sociology Review* 29: 140–148.

Scambler, G. (2022) The elephant in the room: Sayer on social class. In Sanghera, B. and Calder, G. (eds): *Ethics, Economy and Social Science: Dialogues with Andrew Sayer*. London: Routledge.

Scambler, G. (2022a) Let's campaign for a fairer society in the aftermath of COVID-19. *Frontiers of Sociology* 6 (https://doi. org/10.3389/fsoc.2021.789906).

Scambler, G. (2023) *A Critical Realist Theory of Sport*. London: Routledge.

Scambler, G. (2023a) Combining experiential knowledge with scholarship in charting the decline of the National Health Service in England. *Frontiers in Sociology* 8 (https://doi.org/ 10.3389?fsoc.2023.1185487)

Scambler, G. and Kelleher, D. (2006) New social movements: issues of representation and change. *Critical Public Health* 16: 1–13.

Scambler, G. and Scambler, S. (2015) Theorizing health inequalities: the untapped potential of dialectical critical realism. *Social Theory and Health* 13: 340–354.

Scambler, G., Scambler, S. and Speed, E. (2014) Civil society and the Health and Social Care Act in England and Wales: theory and praxis for the twenty-first century. *Social Science and Medicine* 123: 210–216.

Scambler, G., Goodman, B. and Scambler, M. (in press) The potential for muckraking sociology to rebalance the sociological project: putting knowledge under the microscope. In Collyer, F. (ed): *Research Handbook for the Sociology of Knowledge*. Cheltenham: Edward Elgar Publishing.

Scambler, G., Scavarda, A. and Scambler, S. (forthcoming) Whither sociological theory in the health field? *Social Theory and Health*.

Scott, J. (1991) *The Ruling Class*. Cambridge: Polity Press.

Scott, J. (2008) Modes of power and the re-conceptualisation of elites. In Savage, M. and Williams, K. (eds): *Remembering Elites*. Oxford: Blackwell.

SHA NHS Policy Influences Working Group (2023) In Place of Profit. London: SHA.

Short, D. (2010) Cultural genocide and indigenous peoples: a sociological approach. *International Journal of Human Rights* 14: 833–848.

Slater, T. (2014) The myth of 'Broken Britain': welfare reform and the production of ignorance. *Antipode* 46: 948–969.

Smith, R. (2023) Time to ban the word 'prevention'. *British Medical Journal* 382: 2212.

Soper, K. (2023) *Post-Growth Living: For an Alternative Hedonism.* London: Verso.

Stacey, M. (1988) *The Sociology of Health and Healing.* London: Routledge.

Standing, G. (2017) *The Corruption of Capitalism: Why Rentiers Thrive and Work Does Not Pay.* London: Biteback Publishing.

Stedman Jones, G. (2017) *Karl Marx: Greatness and Illusion.* London: Penguin Books.

Steverding, D. (2008) The history of African trypanosomiasis. *Parasites and Vectors* 1: 3.

Stone, J. (2016) Jeremy Hunt co-authored a book calling for the NHS to be replaced with private insurance. *The Independent*, 10 February. Available from: www.independent.co.uk/news/uk/politics/jeremy-hunt-privatise-nhs-tories-privatising-private-insurance-market-replacement-direct-democracy-a6865306.html

Strauss, S. and Mapes, K. (2012) Union power in public utilities: defending worker and consumer health safety. *New Labor Forum* 21: 87–95.

Stuckler, D., Reeves, A., Loopstra, R., Karanikolos, M. and McKee, M. (2017) Austerity and health: the impact in the UK and Europe. *European Journal of Public Health* 27: 18–21.

Thompson, J. (1995) *The Media and Modernity: A Social Theory of the Media.* Cambridge: Polity Press.

Tombs, S. (2020) Home as a site of state-corporate violence: Grenfell Tower, aetiologies and aftermaths. *Howard Journal of Criminal Justice* 59: 120–142.

Townsend, P. and Davidson, N. (eds) (1982) *The Black Report and the Health Divide.* Harmondsworth: Penguin.

UCL News (2023) Covid pandemic disproportionately affected children in BAME families by exacerbating inequalities. *UCL News*, 24 July.

Vankar, P. (2022) US health care expenditure distribution by payer 2015–2022. *Statistica*, 21 November.

Von Heimburg, D., Prilleltensky, I., Ness, O. and Borgunn, Y. (2022) From public health to public good: toward universal wellbeing. *Scandinavian Journal of Public Health* 50: 1062–1070.

Wahl-Jorgensen, K. (2018) Toward a typology of mediated anger: routine coverage of protest and political emotion. *International Journal of Communication* 12: 2017–2087.

Wall, T. (2023) Outsourced care means more children being moved further away – study. *Guardian*, 29 May.

Walsh, D., Dundas, R., McCartney, G., Gibson, M. and Seaman, R. (2022) Bearing the burden of austerity: how do changing mortality rates in the UK compare between men and women? *Epidemiology and Community Health* 76: 1027–1033.

War on Want (2023) Corporate Mercenaries: The Threat of Private Military and Security Companies. London: War on Want (supported by the Campaign Against the Arms Trade).

Ward, H. (2020) We scientists said lock down, but UK politicians refused to listen. *Guardian*, 15 April.

White, K. and Désoulières, S. (2023) Explosive remnants of war: a public health threat. *Lancet* 2: 254–255.

Wilkinson, R. (1996) *Unhealthy Societies: The Afflictions of Inequality*. London: Routledge.

Wilkinson, R. and Pickett, K. (2009) *The Spirit Level: Why More Equal Societies Almost Always Do Better*. London: Allen Lane.

Williams, S. and McKee, M. (2023) How austerity made the UK more vulnerable to COVID. *The Conversation*, 27 July.

World Health Organization (2008) Closing the gap in a generation: health equity through action of social determinants of health: final report of the Commission on Social Determinants of Health. Geneva: WHO.

World Health Organization (2012) What are the social determinants of health? Available from: www.who.int/social_determinants/sdh_definition/en/

World Health Organization (2020) The top ten causes of death. Available from: www.who.int/news-room/fact-sheets/detail/the-top-10-causes-of-death

Wright, E. (2015) *Understanding Class*. London: Verso.

Wright, E. (2016) *Class, Crisis and the State*. London: Verso.

Wright, E. (2019) *How to be an Anti-Capitalist in the Twenty-First Century*. London: Verso.

Index